SUSTAINING
A PLANT-BASED DIET
WITH FILIPINO FOOD

SUSTAINING
A PLANT-BASED DIET
WITH FILIPINO
FOOD

E. VARGAS ALBERTO

Copyright © 2019 by Ely V. Alberto. All rights reserved.

No part of this book may be reproduced, stored in a retrieval system nor transmitted in any form or by any means without prior written permission of the copyright owner.

Edited by Rosemarie Novea
Book design by Anne Alberto
Cover design by indio1571

Images by VectorStock®

ISBN 9781086750607

The material contained in this book is set out in good faith, based on the experiences of the author, as a reference only for those who have already made the decision to try plant-based nutrition on their own. No healing of any kind is being claimed regarding the diet or the food discussed herein.

https://paddygrainpress.com
Email: paddygrainpress@gmail.com

Table of Contents

INTRODUCTION	**11**
1 FILIPINO FOOD AND PLANT-BASED NUTRITION	**14**
The Filipino Taste In Food	14
Adapting The Food To Plant-Based Nutrition	17
Food Sourcing And Preparation	21
Cooking Equipment, Tools And Gadgets	22
2 ESSENTIAL FOOD ITEMS & SUPPLEMENT	**26**
Focus On Brown Rice	26
Boiling Brown Rice	27
Toasting Brown Rice	28
Legumes	28
Seeds	29
Nuts	30
Oats	30
Green Vegetables	31
Vitamin B12	31
3 RECIPES AND COOKING NOTES	**33**
NOTES ON MEASUREMENTS	34
Boiled Brown Rice	35
Turmeric Brown Rice	36
Brown Rice with Quinoa	37
Brown Rice Brínghe	38
USING SPICE MIXES	40
Brown Rice Arroz Caldo	40

SEAWEED-HOISIN FISH SAUCE SUBSTITUTE 42
Toasted Brown Rice 42
USING FROZEN PEAS 43
Staple Bowl 44
REDUCING THE WATER CONTENT OF
  FIRM TOFU 45
Tofu Bisték 46
Crispy-Fried Tofu with Vinegar Dip 47
Green Beans with Tofu Gisádo 48
Tofu Paksíw with Lily Blossoms 49
Bok Choy and Tofu Gisádo 50
Tofu with Garlic Leaves Gisádo 51
USING BANANA LEAVES FOR
  PARCEL COOKING 52
Spicy Tofu Pináis 52
Bitter Gourd with Black Beans Gisádo 53
Kale Chips 54
Kale and White Bean Dip 55
BINDING MINCED INGREDIENTS
  WITHOUT EGGS 56
Tofu-Taro Siomai 57
USING TEXTURED VEGETABLE PROTEIN 59
Tápa Bits Toppings 59
Meatless Longganísa 61
Picadillo with Sweet Potatoes and Sabá 62
Stir-Fried Mixed Vegetables 63
BLANCHING VEGETABLES WITH
  SALTED WATER 65
Lumpiyâ Plate 65
Lumpiyâng Príto 67
Mango Cucumber Ensaladá 68
Kale Quinoa Ensaladá 69
Ókoy 70
SUBSTITUTING VINEGARS FOR
  FLAVOR VARIETY 72
Pinakbét 72
Stir-Fried Pinakbét Vegetables 74

Sótanghón Gisádo	76
USING SÓTANGHÓN OR GLASS NOODLES	77
Sótanghón with Bottle Gourd	77
Laksá-Laksá	78
USING AND CLEANING FRESH BANANA BLOSSOMS	80
Sótanghón Hot Pot	80
Sótanghón with Sponge Gourd	81
Sótanghón Asado Noodles	82
USING TRADITIONAL FRUIT VEGETABLES	84
Banana Blossoms with Sótanghón	84
Oyster Mushroom Gisádo	85
Eggplant Iníhaw with Coconut Milk	86
Cheesy Pimiento Spread	87
Kangkóng Adóbo	88
Snake Beans Adóbo	88
Bamboo Shoot Adóbo	89
Mung Beans with Bitter Gourd Leaves Gisádo	90
Bamboo Shoot Gisádo	92
Cabbage and Carrots Gisádo	93
Mushroom and Bok Choy Gisádo	94
Tahô with Tapioca Pearls	95
Eggplant Bisték	95
Leafy Greens with Stir-fry Sauce	96
Laíng	97
Ensaladáng Pilipino	99
Pico De Gallo	100
Mung Bean Sprouts Ensaladá	101
Carrots and Green Beans Ensaladá	102
Cauliflower Ensaladá	103
Bitter Gourd Tomato Ensaladá	104
BOILING SWEET POTATOES	105
USING FROZEN CORN KERNELS	106
Oven-Roasted Vegetables with Garden Ensaladá	106
Barbecue Broad Beans and Chickpeas	108

Lima Beans Sinigáng	109
Lima Beans with Sweet Potato Gisádo	111
USING CANNED BEANS	112
Canned Beans Snacks	113
Tomato Basil Pesto	114
White Beans with Tomato Pesto	115
Pasta with Tomato Pesto	116
Pesto Pizza	116
Roasted Lima Beans Snack	119
Ampalayá Smoothie	120
Creamed Corn-Split Pea Suwám	121
Lentil and Sweet Potato Bóla-Bóla	122
Braised Carrots and Chayote	123
Spaghetti with Sweet Tomato Sauce	124
Cheesy Oats Púto	126
Salabát	127
Tápa Bits Pináis with Turmeric Rice	128
Mung Beans with Maple Soy Milk	129
Banana Oats Maruyà	130
Meatless Longganísa Pináis	132
Oven-Roasted Vegetables with Beans	132
Mixed Beans with Bell Pepper Gisádo	133
Squash Soup with Moringa Leaves	134
Quick Banana Blossom Sísig	136
Red Cabbage Coleslaw with Atsára Pickling Solution	137
Breadfruit and Green Beans in Coconut Cream	138
Vegetable Tinóla	139
FREEZE-DRYING TOFU	140
Tofu Karékaré	141
Tofu Apritáda	143
Tofu Skewers	144
Banana Blossom Litsón Paksíw	145
Freeze-dried Tofu Eskabétse	147
Tofu Sísig	148

ACKNOWLEDGEMENT	**151**
DEDICATION	**152**
BIBLIOGRAPHY	**153**
RECIPE INDEX	**155**
ABOUT THE AUTHOR	**159**

INTRODUCTION

The exclusion of animal-derived products from dietary consumption may be a common and unifying idea for everyone on a plant-based diet. However, the choice of a staple cuisine for those who have just made the decision and are only about to start with the diet change will definitely vary among individuals.

Depending on their appreciation of the food traditions from other cultures, there will be a fraction who will find it relatively easier to adjust to the diet change. Their openness will be the key to their acceptance of an entirely different set of food ways.

Another part from more selective cultures, on the other hand, will be looking to improvise to accommodate the newly adapted, less-inclusive diet. For them, the familiar food tastes from their own cultural backgrounds will be an obvious preference.

It is on these preferences, these specific tastes in food that a transition diet needs to be based on to make the diet change more acceptable and appealing and, therefore, more sustainable as a permanent endeavor.

Making a plant-based diet an essential part of a healthy lifestyle is attainable as a long-term goal with a stronger foundation, when beneficial health gains from the diet change would have been evident.

The immediate goal upon starting the diet shift, however, should be sustainability. That is, familiarizing and getting used to the diet without reverting to the consumption of meat, seafood and dairy products.

This book is for those who prefer the food that Filipinos love to eat for their usual fare on regular and uneventful days.

We have collated several home-style recipes in this volume and these are plainly presented. The procedures are as simple as could be workable for those who may want to take charge of the preparation and cooking of their own food or at least supervise it.

The goal of this book is to make the diet change less of an effort and more of an enjoyable undertaking that people do for themselves as it seeks to minimize the guesswork out of the leap to a plant-based diet.

Whatever their motivation for the diet change may be, readers are encouraged to consult their own trusted medical professionals before making the decision to change from an omnivorous diet to purely plant-based nutrition.

They should also be aware of their own food allergies and other health issues and problems as they relate to the food they decide to try. This is strongly urged as regards the recipes that are discussed in this book.

Because we have different needs pertaining to our individual health, we need to be responsible for our own health and well-being. When in doubt, we should always defer to the wisdom and heed the advice of our doctors.

1

FILIPINO FOOD AND PLANT-BASED NUTRITION

FILIPINO FOOD AND PLANT-BASED NUTRITION

THE FILIPINO TASTE IN FOOD

Philippine cuisine is based on seafood and meat products. Even the few that we classify as vegetable dishes contain some bits of fish, shrimps, meat or poultry mixed in to boost the taste of vegetables.

Due to its topography and the abundance of marine life in mythic, unpolluted waters, the main source of protein in the islands had traditionally been fish and other seafood.

Condiments that were developed early on were sourced from salty waters. Not surprisingly though, fish sauce (*patís*), shrimp paste (*bagoóng alamáng*), the more diluted *bagoóng isdâ* and even sea salt (*asín*) are still the preferred flavorings for saltiness up to the present times.

Aside from these, either fried or roasted fish were usually added to enhance the taste of either braised or boiled dishes. This is all the more evident in today's cooking especially when vegetable dishes are cooked in boiling broth.

Our ancestors learned the process of making fish sauce from Chinese traders and sojourners who used to bring along their food when they visited the islands. The production of *bagoóng* was an indigenous technology that was probably invented to make use of the fish and krill by-products from making *patís*.

Among the early contributions of the Chinese to our cooking were soy sauce or *toyò* along with tofu or *tókwa*, which were both derived from soybeans. These ingredients had been part of our cooking for several centuries before Europeans arrived.

FILIPINO FOOD AND PLANT-BASED NUTRITION

Because they are plant-based, they have attained greater significance to our purpose-driven diet change in our own time.

Antonio Pigafetta, the official chronicler of the Fernão de Magalhães expedition, had provided us with a glimpse of the way our ancestors cooked their food when the *conquistadores* surveyed the islands. While the natives were noted as processing products like vinegar, wine and coconut milk from the coconut trees that lined the landscape, cooking was obviously basic and rudimentary.

Magalhães and his men were served, as esteemed visitors, meat and fish with rice—not a single vegetable dish in the forty-one days that they stayed on. All of the dishes were cooked with the use of simple methods like broiling on hot coals and boiling in water to bring out the juices of meat and fish.

The cooking procedures with the use of oil which included sautéing with garlic and onions were introduced to the islanders by the Spaniards during the colonial period. This is the reason why terms like frying (*príto*, from the Spanish word *frito*) and sautéing (*gisá*, from the Spanish root word *guisar*) do not have equivalent words in our local languages.

During this period, Philippine food substantially changed. Focus has shifted more to meat and poultry. Dishes like tinola, afritada, caldereta, mechado, menudo, estofado, pochero, lengua, embutido, hamonado, asado and many others were developed to please the distinctive tastes of the ruling *peninsulares*—elite Spaniards from the Iberian Peninsula.

These food items would later be showcased and served during annual religious feasts. Eventually, they would become the food of the more affluent strata of society and, much later on, were integrated into the mainstream of the culinary culture.

SUSTAINING A PLANT-BASED DIET WITH FILIPINO FOOD

To simplify our scope on the subject of Filipino cooking for purposes of this book, we shall concentrate on the Spanish and Chinese influences on the cuisine, which are arguably the greater, more lasting legacies. But if there had to be just a single cooking skill with an impact that had been imparted to our people by foreigners, it would have to be the procedure on how to do a sauté with the use of garlic and onion.

Here we have to underscore the importance of the cooking procedure—particularly its potential in the infusion of the unique flavors of the sauté bulbs, rhizome and fruit vegetable to perk-up the taste of dishes.

To be fair, there had been numerous important influences to the food culture in conjunction with the Chinese influences. There were the Arabs and the island neighbors from the maritime realm which comprised the more extensive universe of our ancestors for both trade and social interaction in ancient times. That phase in history certainly left indelible marks particularly in regional cooking.

In the same manner, there were also influences on the food culture after the Spanish rule in the more recent American occupation of the nation. It is worth emphasizing also that, in contrast with more conservative Spaniards, the Americans had been less proprietary in transferring knowledge and skills which altered the lifestyle significantly, the food culture included.

It had been said often and even immortalized in literature that in cooking, Filipinos improve everything with onions and garlic. Among the basic skills that a Filipino parent teaches her offspring in the kitchen would have to include this irreplaceable cooking procedure.

We can see the sauté with the use of garlic and onions and also ginger, which is endemic to Island Southeast Asia, and

FILIPINO FOOD AND PLANT-BASED NUTRITION

the likewise introduced fruit-vegetable, tomato, in a number of our dishes. Our thinking is dishes that were already being cooked prior to the introduction of the bulb sauté had been transformed to include this cooking procedure.

A good example of this is the way an ordinary home cook would prepare the Ilocano-created vegetable dish, the classic called pinakbét at the present time.

The dish is traditionally cooked by braising with *bagoóng monámon* (anchovy) and heated well in an earthen pot to 'shrink'—the defining characteristic that gave the dish its name—the mixture of vegetables. But because a lot of our dishes are started off as a sauté, this very distinct dish too will be cooked in the same way by the ordinary home cook.

We see it too in the way we cook stir-fried food. The cooking method involves pre-heating the wok to very high heat before we add in the oil, which is quickly followed by the sauté ingredients. More often than not, we have to undergo the sauté ritual of browning the garlic, softening the onions and ginger until they are fragrant and waiting for the tomatoes to break down before proceeding.

The sauté, in combination with a choice of condiments has, the way we see it, evolved to be the premier taste of Filipino food.

ADAPTING THE FOOD TO PLANT-BASED NUTRITION

The initial step in preparing Filipino food as a viable and staple food base to use in plant-based nutrition is to identify and enumerate all-vegetable dishes from a listing of mainstream dishes.

SUSTAINING A PLANT-BASED DIET WITH FILIPINO FOOD

This slim list will comprise your go-to food when imagination fails and food choices point back to food that are peppered with animal-derived products.

We start off with ensaladás, which are either blanched or lightly-boiled vegetables like sweet potato tops, kangkóng leaves, chayote tops, squash tops, some greens from our Asian neighbors that are available at the fresh vegetables market. Yes, even some seaweed known in Filipino as *latô*.

Usually dressed with something sour like tomatoes or vinegar together with salt, fish sauce or shrimp paste, there are a lot of variations, especially in the farming countryside. Just do away with shrimp paste and fish sauce. Soy sauce, especially the lighter kind, or tamari will be a good alternative. When out of choices there is always the old dependable sea salt.

We can also count on modifying mixed vegetable-meat, vegetable-poultry and vegetable-seafood dishes with purely vegetable ingredients to augment our food list. We could perhaps cook these mixed vegetable dishes without the added bits of fish, shrimps, meat and poultry from such dishes as *dinengdéng*, *láswa*, *munggó gisádo*, *abráw* et al but also cooked with plant-based condiments.

What would give us more extensive choices for variety in our dishes, however, would be turning our traditional seafood, meat and poultry dishes into plant-based variations through ingredient substitution. Here we might utilize more high protein substitutes like tofu and pulses or we can just be creative in coming up with ingredient combinations.

Let us be mindful though in our ingredient substitution to achieve a plant-based alternative that it is our own food we are cooking. Taste, of course, will be of primary importance and never mind that picture-worthy depiction of your food for some audience. Food do not always look good but they do have to please the taste buds all the time.

FILIPINO FOOD AND PLANT-BASED NUTRITION

When faced with a situation when we cannot seem to find the correct formula to replicate a taste, let us try doing it the other way altogether. We might be surprised at the result.

Let's take the cooking of mung bean soup as an example. Everyone knows that this protein-rich soup is best seasoned with seafood condiments like fish sauce or shrimp paste which are, of course, animal-derived. Who can figure out why the distinct green and grainy taste of mung bean goes well with the taste of the sea? Well, it just does.

There are times as well when we feel that our plant-based condiment concoctions seem to have achieved that similar taste when tried out of a spoon. It turns out later it doesn't translate well when they are used to season our favorite vegetable dishes.

Our own solution for this is to do away with the seafood condiment taste by turning to salt and adding in more vegetables like green chilli peppers for flavor, starchy pump-kin for a bit of sweetness and other available vegetables with agreeable tastes like cauliflower, sponge gourd etc. and leafy green vegetables like baby spinach leaves. If a dish can't be as tasty, then let's compensate for it by making it more nutritious.

Eliminating meat, poultry, seafood and dairy from our array of ingredients means we will be losing out not just a major source of dietary protein. We will also be missing out on a unique element of flavor that is responsible for the desirable taste of traditional dishes. Meat, admittedly, can be a difficult ingredient to replace primarily because of its taste. So, how do we go about it?

In plant-based cooking, creativity and innovation are tools of crucial importance. We can remedy the problems of protein

SUSTAINING A PLANT-BASED DIET WITH FILIPINO FOOD

alternatives and the problem of taste or flavors by doing the following:

- innovate by replacing fleshy animal protein with plant protein from food such as **brown rice**; **legumes** i.e. peanuts, pulses such as beans, lentils and peas; **seeds** like quinoa, chia, pumpkin seeds, sesame seeds and flax seeds; **nuts** such as cashew nuts, almonds and pine nuts; **oats** and other whole-food; and **green vegetables** such as spinach, kale, broccoli and bok choy.

- innovate by using **vegetable stocks** that were developed to approximate the flavors of meat and poultry stock. Some leading brands carry these special vegetable stocks, both in liquid and powdered form, and are prominently labeled on the packaging as **beef-style**, **chicken-style**, etc.

- innovate by using **high-protein meat substitutes** that we trust to fulfill our requirements and that we are confident in adding to our cooking. Scan the market for available options, including conveniently packaged meat-like products like sausages, hotdogs, nuggets, etc. For the recipes on the following pages, we will be using **tofu** and **textured vegetable protein**.

- innovate by using **vegetarian** or **vegan flavorings** like **stir-fry sauces**, **fish sauce substitutes**, **shrimp paste substitutes** that will go well with vegetable cookery. Here is where the internet can come in handy. You'll be surprised about the range of options when you search online. Identify two or three suppliers that serve your area and try out their products. Reading the reviews from previous customers could be invaluable.

FILIPINO FOOD AND PLANT-BASED NUTRITION

SOURCING AND PREPARATION

It is always desirable to start changes regarding lifestyle, particularly as regards diet, with the whole family complete with their support. But if that is not at all possible and the family cannot join you, taking charge of your own food is one sure way to put the diet change on track, but family support will still be nice. Just the caring reminders from really concerned people that count can sometimes spell the difference between quitting and striving on.

Be aware that during the first days, possibly weeks, on an all-plant diet you might feel hungry more often than when you've had meat and poultry for your main meals. It is nothing unhealthy and is perfectly normal, which could only mean the body is adjusting to the change. Always have something on hand though for situations like these. Your favorite fruits like apples, bananas, pears or cut vegetables like carrot sticks or celery sticks may just be your life-saver, so to speak.

Begin by setting apart one's piece of the household's shared food storage, which include the pantry and refrigerator, for your supplies. Here, you can store all canned, dried, fresh and frozen vegetable products that you don't regularly buy for the entire family.

- Familiarize yourself with the wet market, fresh food section of the supermarket or a fruits and vegetables market. Remember that you exert extra effort and go out of your way to get hold of fresh produce so don't let it go to waste. As a general rule in planning your meals, fresh fruits and vegetables should be consumed first.

- Scan the frozen section of the supermarket for choice products you can buy just in case you run out of fresh

21

SUSTAINING A PLANT-BASED DIET WITH FILIPINO FOOD

options from your supply storage. Green peas, corn kernels, sweet potato fries etc. are just some of the choices you can get from this section. This is also where most supermarkets store and stock their vegan and vegetarian meat substitute products. Always read the labels and watch out for some ingredients you may not be aware of are animal-derived. If in doubt, do some research. Google is your friend.

- Canned vegetable products and pulses are another convenient way to ensure you don't run out of sup-plies. Stock up on canned products like baked beans and an assortment of pulses like red kidney beans, white beans, pinto beans, butter beans, brown lentils and a lot more others. Vegetable products like, bamboo shoots, young corn, jackfruit, breadfruit, water chestnuts, mushrooms, etc. also come in cans. Some of the recipes included in the later section are based on these canned products. You can find canned vegetables from the supermarket, Asian Food Stores and even some fresh fruits and vegetable stores.

COOKING EQUIPMENT, TOOLS AND GADGETS

To be able to cook the recipes in the following pages we shall need a list of simple equipment, tools and gadgets that you most probably already have. Those that we find to be particularly useful and convenient to use are highlighted in block letters. With the exception of the big equipment like kitchen stove or cook top and oven, it will be a good idea to get these useful cooking basics by the set as we usually need them from time to time.

- Kitchen Stove or Cook top, a gas or LPG-fueled one will be convenient when cooking recipes with several shifting heat settings.
- Oven

FILIPINO FOOD AND PLANT-BASED NUTRITION

- Charcoal Barbecue
- Oven Toaster
- Rice Cooker, usually comes with a measuring cup equivalent to a standard half cup.
- Blender
- Food Processor
- Cooking Pots
- Stock Pots
- Steamer set
- Frying Pans, choose a non-stick brand.
- Wok, choose a non-stick brand.
- Ceramic Mixing Bowls
- Plastic Mixing Bowls
- Metal Mixing Bowls
- Measuring Cups
- Graduated Liquid Measuring Cups
- Measuring Spoons
- Culture and Enzyme Measuring Spoons, with small fraction measurements for tad (¼ tsp), dash (⅛ tsp), pinch ($1/16$ tsp), smidgen ($1/32$ tsp) and drop ($1/64$ tsp).
- Wire Sieves
- Colanders
- Tongs
- Spatula
- **Salad Spinner**, for drying washed fruits and vegetables.
- **Papaya Salad Grater**, for making quick long strips of fleshy and starchy vegetables.
- **Fruit and Vegetable Peeler**, for quick and convenient peeling of fruits and vegetables.
- **Rubber Scraper**, for use during quick-movement stir-frying, also for scraping batter-like mixes like tempura. The rubber scraper is a baking utensil that is more convenient to use than a ladle or turner.

2

ESSENTIAL FOOD ITEMS AND SUPPLEMENT

SUSTAINING A PLANT-BASED DIET WITH FILIPINO FOOD

ESSENTIAL FOOD ITEMS AND SUPPLEMENT

BROWN RICE

Unmilled rice which we currently find in the market under such labels as brown rice, black rice, red rice and other similar types of pigmented rice grains are wholefood. They are intermediate products that increasingly became more common apparently as a response to market demand.

Known as *pinawà* in Filipino, unmilled rice is the whole grain where only the inedible chaff or the husk (*ipá*) of the paddy grain (*pálay*) is removed.

The market names are determined by the color variations of the rice grain's outer layer. Jasmine rice, for example, will have a brown outer color after the rice husk is removed so it will be labeled as brown rice. *Sinandómeng* will have a red outer color so it will be sold as red rice, and so on.

Almost every variety of rice, from basmati to the uncommon rice varieties with naturally low glycemic indices, can be produced or consumed as unmilled rice.

For purposes of this book, the widely-used term brown rice shall be used to mean any type of unmilled rice no matter what the variety or pigment may be.

Brown rice retains the nutritious parts of the grain that are usually removed during the milling process. These include the fiber-rich bran—called *darák* in Filipino—which is also a good source of micronutrients and minerals.

ESSENTIAL FOOD ITEMS AND SUPPLEMENT

Another by-product of rice milling called *binlíd*, in Filipino, the rice germ which is rich in polyunsaturated fats is also retained in brown rice.

Peripherally flanking the endosperm, the aleurone layer—host to a significant amount of the grain's protein—is also intact in brown rice.

These healthful ingredients being part of the nourishment we get from eating brown rice should justify the recent public perception that gave rise to the increased popularity of the cereal.

Boiling Brown Rice

Because of the presence of these layers that effectively seal the rice grain's starchy endosperm, the cooking of brown rice by boiling is slightly different from boiling white rice or polished rice.

During boiling, the absorption of water is substantially inhibited by these parts of the rice grain that are otherwise removed in the milling process.

The absorption of water by the grain is an important facet in boiling rice. When heated, the retained moisture causes the expansion of the grain to attain that desirable fluffy quality.

Excess water in improperly cooked brown rice settles at the bottom of the cooking pot. This results in mushy later plates of cooked rice. Excess water, combined with adverse keeping properties of the retained parts in brown rice, also causes easy spoilage especially during the warmer months.

When boiling brown rice, one needs to keep watch and alternately cover and uncover the lid of the rice cooker. This is to ensure that the cooking rice retains just the proper amount

SUSTAINING A PLANT-BASED DIET WITH FILIPINO FOOD

of water while also making sure there is sufficient heat to allow the rice grains to absorb the required amount of moisture to rise optimally.

Toasting Brown Rice

Due to the same reason that it cannot absorb too much water, cooked brown rice also cannot take in too much oil or salt when cooking it by toasting. This is why it cannot be fried as one would regular or polished rice.

Left-over brown rice is best toasted in a wok, which may be lightly lined with oil spray. Unlike starchy white rice, however, brown rice is not sticky and is easily stirred about on the wok. When stored in the refrigerator before toasting, the grains readily come apart when crumbled.

During toasting, heat should be kept high while the grains are continuously stirred around to make all sides touch the very hot surface of the wok. This way, the grains could form a crust quickly without drying up the inner part.

LEGUMES

Legumes are plants that bear seeded fruits which are enclosed in a pod. In the Philippine setting, popular legumes are trees like the tamarind (*sampálok*) and the *ípil-ípil*, shrubs like the mung bean (*munggó*) and peanut (*maní*), vines like string-beans (*sitáw*), hyacinth bean (*bátaw*), lima bean (*patani*), winged bean (*sigarílyas*) and the only vine that is cultivated for its tuber root in the bean family, the Mexican yam bean or jicama (*singkamás*).

The string varieties are widely useful in Philippine cookery and are regularly added to improve the protein quality of mixed vegetable dishes. But of all the wide array of pulses—

ESSENTIAL FOOD ITEMS AND SUPPLEMENT

legumes that are cultivated because of the high protein content of their dry seeds—we are only familiar with lima beans and mung beans.

We may see some of the more popular beans like the red kidney beans and white beans being cooked in syrup and added in popular refreshments like the *haló-halò* but the Philippine cooking scene is missing out on this excellent source of plant protein.

In plant-based cooking, dry seed beans, peas and lentils take a prominent place as an important source of plant protein, being regarded in their unprocessed forms as direct replacement to animal protein. They can be added in soup vegetable dishes, stir-fried vegetables, sauced and served singly as a meal, added in salads, sautéed as added protein with other vegetables, baked dry as a snack item, etc.

SEEDS

Another plant food item that is not regarded well in Philippine cooking is the seed.

The word seed denotes a broad botanical classification that includes grains, cereals, legumes and nuts. For purposes of this book, however, we shall refer to seeds that, due to their tiny size, are often dismissed as *pagkáing-íbon* or bird-seeds by the uninformed. These include the pseudo-cereals chia and quinoa, the cypsela sunflower seed, flaxseed or linseed and sesame seed (*lingá*).

Along with nuts and with the exception of quinoa which has a negligible fat content, seeds are recommended sources of dietary fats to replace the restriction of animal fat in a plant-based diet. They are also excellent sources of plant protein.

SUSTAINING A PLANT-BASED DIET WITH FILIPINO FOOD

They can be easily added to smoothies and healthful cereal dishes especially because they have an agreeable taste and would blend well with different flavors.

NUTS

Another excellent source of plant protein that are almost comparable to their own carbohydrate content, nuts are also very good sources of healthy fats. They are nearly the big brother of seeds because of their make-up and nutritional value and are more widely used especially in baking and patisserie.

In Philippine cooking, we are familiar with the cashew (*kasúy*) nut and the Bicol-region endemic pilì nut.

In plant-based cooking, nuts are valuable for their use as thickeners in sauces like pesto, added for texture in stir-fried vegetable dishes and even in making nut milks, plant-based yoghurts and plant-based mayonnaise.

OATS

Aside from having high dietary and soluble fibers, oat is the only cereal grain with a protein content that is comparable to pulses. A host of micronutrients and minerals complete its exceptional nutrient profile.

In the Philippines, oats are among the food items that were popularized during the American regime. It is usually eaten as a breakfast fare or as an in-between meal or snacks.

In a plant-based diet, oats can be used as a flour substitute or as an alternative thickener in various sauces. Used in appropriate amounts, it can even work to improve the texture

ESSENTIAL FOOD ITEMS AND SUPPLEMENT

of baked products, particularly when a crunchy finish is desired.

To use as oat flour, you simply pulverize the cereal in small amounts using an ordinary blender.

GREEN VEGETABLES

Except when used in salads, green leafy vegetables are not really maximized in Philippine cooking. They are usually added as a finishing touch to adorn soupy meat dishes or stews. The limited range include bok choy (*pétsay*), chinese cabbage, water spinach (*kangkóng*) and sweet potato tops (*talbós*).

Although not as prolific a source of protein as the other food ingredients mentioned in this section, leafy greens should be given attention because they are a rich source of micronutrients and minerals.

We may want to add to our regular fare some raw salads with dark green kale and baby spinach leaves. We took the liberty of adding some recipes that highlight these green leafy vegetables. While we are on the subject of suggestion, we might also want to try if we could get used to having some raw onions with our salads as well.

VITAMIN B12: THE SUPPLEMENT WE NEED

Because only food that come from animal sources contain this important micronutrient, people on an exclusive plant-based diet will require regular supplementation. Fortunately, the human body needs it in minute amounts only. The daily recommended intake of 2.4 mcg may be derived from a B-complex vitamin or most multivitamins.

SUSTAINING A PLANT-BASED DIET WITH FILIPINO FOOD

Vitamin B12 is unique among the water-soluble group of micronutrients since it is the only kind that has the characteristic to get stored in the body. Still, this is not reason enough to be complacent as we need to take the precaution to supplement our stores of the vitamin seriously.

Vitamin B12 promotes the formation and regeneration of red blood cells.

Vitamin B12 is also often added in vegan products like sausages, nuggets and other meat substitutes. It is also available in sufficient quantities from the vegan cheese substitute called nutritional yeast flakes.

3

RECIPES AND COOKING NOTES

RECIPES AND
COOKING NOTES

NOTES ON MEASUREMENTS

Standard cup and spoon measurements are indicative quantities and have been included specifically to aid the cook in making practical calculations such as how much ingredients to prepare and cook and for how many people, etc.

Metric quantities may vary between recipes especially among differently-sized vegetables and other ingredients.

Whenever possible, please use the metric quantities included in the recipes in your cooking for best results. This practice will also ensure consistency of outcome every time you cook the same recipes.

RECIPES AND COOKING NOTES

BOILED BROWN RICE

Cooking rice by boiling is the traditional Filipino way of cooking the cereal. In this and following recipes, the use of a rice cooker is recommended although brown rice may also be cooked in a heavy-set pot over low heat using the same rice-to-water proportion. If recipe instructions are followed, cooked brown rice will not retain any excess water.

Ingredients:

2 cups, dry	BROWN RICE	400 g
4 cups	WATER	1 L

(Serves 4)

Procedures:

1. In a wire sieve, rinse the rice grains in running water and drain.
2. Combine the rice and water in the pot holder of the rice cooker with a quick stir, cover and turn the rice cooker on.
3. Wait until the pot begins to boil briskly and for steam to get heavy to lift the lid off and let it cook uncovered until no more liquid is visible on top.
4. When the steam has settled at the level of the grains, put the lid back on to let the cooking rice absorb moisture and rise some more.
5. Lift the lid off and leave the rice cooker uncovered for another five minutes when the rice cooker setting has shifted to WARM to let more steam escape.

35

SUSTAINING A PLANT-BASED DIET WITH FILIPINO FOOD

6. Put the lid back on and wait another five minutes to make sure the rice is well cooked through before turning off the rice cooker.

TURMERIC BROWN RICE

Turmeric powder is a rhizome powder that has been traditionally used as a flavoring for white rice especially in the northernmost islands in the home country where the turmeric crop is usually grown. The flavoring powder works just as well with brown rice.

Ingredients:

2 cups, dry	BROWN RICE	400 g
1 tsp	TURMERIC POWDER	5 g
1 tsp	TABLE SALT, optional	5 g
4 cups	WATER	1 L

(Serves 4)

Procedures:

1. Dissolve the turmeric powder and salt in water and place in the rice cooker pot.
2. In a wire sieve, rinse the rice grains in running water and drain.
3. Combine the rice with the liquid in the pot holder of the rice cooker with a quick stir, cover and turn the rice cooker on.
4. Wait until the pot begins to boil briskly and for steam to get heavy to take the lid off and let the rice cook uncovered until no more liquid is visible on top.
5. Put the lid back on when the steam has settled at the level of the grains to let the cooking rice absorb moisture and rise some more.

RECIPES AND COOKING NOTES

6. Lift the lid off and leave the rice cooker uncovered for another five minutes when the rice cooker setting shifts to WARM to let more steam escape.
7. Put the lid back on and wait for another five minutes to make sure the rice is well-cooked and turn the rice cooker off.

BROWN RICE WITH QUINOA

Brown rice and quinoa are two grains that complement each other and combine very well. During cooking, the excess water that cannot be absorbed by the brown rice is easily taken up by the quinoa. This results in a perfectly cooked and fluffy pot of staple every time, aside from being fortified nutritionally.

Ingredients:

1 cup, dry	BROWN RICE	200 g
1 cup, dry	QUINOA	180 g
4 cups	WATER	1 L

(Serves 3)

Procedures:

1. In a wire sieve, combine the brown rice and quinoa and sift dry to rid the grains of bits of hulls from the quinoa.
2. Rinse in running water and drain.
3. Combine the rice and quinoa with water in the pot holder of the rice cooker with a quick stir, cover and turn the rice cooker on.
4. Keep the grains covered at all time while cooking.
5. When the rice cooker setting shifts to WARM, leave for five to ten minutes more before turning off the rice cooke

37

SUSTAINING A PLANT-BASED DIET WITH FILIPINO FOOD

BROWN RICE BRÍNGHE

Brínghe is the Kapampángan variation of the Spanish dish paella. The dish is similarly called in Cebuano cooking while the Ilonggo call it arroz a la valenciana. This plant-based variation minimally aimed for the rich and subtly-spiced rice to provide a contrast to the simply flavored vegetable viands.

Turmeric Rice Base

Ingredients:

3 cups, dry	BROWN RICE	600 g
4 cups	WATER	1 L
2 cups	COCONUT CREAM	500 ml
2 tsp	TURMERIC POWDER	10 g
1 tsp	SALT, optional	5 g

(Serves 6)

Procedures:

1. In a water container, combine water and coconut cream and dissolve the turmeric powder and salt.
2. In a wire sieve, rinse the rice grains in running water and drain well.
3. Mix the rinsed rice inside the rice cooker pot and add the turmeric water.
4. Stir well using a rubber scraper or spatula to combine and turn the rice cooker on.
5. When the pot begins to boil briskly and the steam to get heavy, take the lid off the rice cooker.
6. Leave the lid off just until water can barely be seen on top.
7. Put the lid back on to let the cooking rice absorb more

RECIPES AND COOKING NOTES

moisture and rise.
8. When the rice cooker turns to WARM wait for five minutes before turning it off.

Viands

Ingredients:

1 cup	CHICKPEAS, cooked	175 g
1 pc	RED BELL PEPPER or capsicum, roasted and chopped	180 g
1 pc	GREEN BELL PEPPER or capsicum, roasted and chopped	180 g
3 pc	EGGPLANTS, roasted and chopped	200 g
½ cup	RAISINS	90 g
½ cup, dry	TEXTURED VEGETABLE PROTEIN	42 g
1 pc	VEGETABLE STOCK CUBE, chicken-style	10 g
½ cup	WATER	120 ml
½ tsp	SALT	2.5 g
1 tsp	SRIRACHA SAUCE	5 ml
½ pack	CALDERETA MIX, pre-packed spice mix	25 g
1 tbsp	SUNFLOWER OIL	15 ml
1 pc	RED ONION, chopped finely	120 g

Procedures:

1. In a small cooking pot, dissolve the vegetable stock cube in water.
2. Add the salt and sriracha sauce and cook to medium heat until the mixture begins to boil.
3. Turn off the heat and add the textured vegetable protein. Cool.
4. In a large non-stick wok, heat the oil to medium heat.
5. Sauté the onions just until they change colors.
6. Add the caldereta mix and stir-fry for another minute.

SUSTAINING A PLANT-BASED DIET WITH FILIPINO FOOD

7. Add the hydrated vegetable protein, bell peppers, egg-plants and raisins.
8. Stir-fry for five minutes until everything is blended well and is evenly distributed. Turn off heat.
9. In the same wok, add the cooked turmeric rice to the viands and mix thoroughly.

USING SPICE MIXES

Using ready mixed spice combinations is a convenient way to add flavor to plant-based food.

Spice mixes are usually a combination of powdered spices and flavorings that approximate a certain type of cooking such as Mexican Chipotle, Moroccan Spices, Cajun Spices among others. They are also available in local flavors like caldereta, adobo, guisado, etc.

Spice mixes, being preserved in powdered form, may or may not contain preservatives. Choose ones that are free from these additives just to be safe.

BROWN RICE ARROZ CALDO

Arroz caldo is the Filipino variation of the Chinese congee where rice is cooked in broth until it attains the consistency of porridge. It is usually cooked with chicken and pork or beef innards as main ingredients. As a protein substitute we added split peas to the brown rice base in this plant-based variation of the dish.

Ingredients:

½ cup, dry BROWN RICE   100 g

RECIPES AND COOKING NOTES

½ cup	YELLOW SPLIT PEAS, soaked for one hour	100 g
1 tbsp	SUNFLOWER OIL	15 ml
4 cloves	GARLIC, minced	16 g
1 tbsp	GINGER, slivered	20 g
8 cups	WATER	2 L
3 pc	VEGETABLE STOCK CUBES, chicken-style	30 g
Dash of	COARSELY GROUND BLACK PEPPER	
To taste,	FISH SAUCE SUBSTITUTE, recipe on the next page	
¼ cup	FRIED GARLIC, to garnish	24 g
½ cup	GREEN ONIONS, finely chopped, to garnish	30 g
1 large pc	RED ONION, chopped	120 g

(Serves 4)

Procedures:

1. In a wire sieve, rinse the mixed brown rice and split peas in running water and drain thoroughly.
2. In a large cooking pot, heat the oil to medium heat and sauté the garlic until golden brown in color.
3. Add the onions and ginger just until they change colors.
4. Add the combined brown rice and peas and stir in the sauté until everything is well coated with the oil.
5. Add the water and vegetable stock cubes and bring to a boil.
6. When the pot reaches a rolling boil, reduce heat to simmer and add the fish sauce substitute starting with a tablespoon of the condiment.
7. Mix the cooking rice and peas occasionally, making sure nothing sticks to the bottom of the pot.
8. Continue cooking until the brown rice has broken down and the peas are well cooked.
9. Serve with fried garlic and chopped green onions

SUSTAINING A PLANT-BASED DIET WITH FILIPINO FOOD

SEAWEED-HOISIN FISH SAUCE SUBSTITUTE

Ingredients:

¾ cup	BOILING WATER	200 ml
2 tbsp	DRIED SEAWEED STRIPS, KELP	10 g
2 tsp	SEA SALT	14 g
1 tsp	HOISIN SAUCE	5 g

Procedures:

Place the seaweed strips in a small bowl and pour the boiling water, making sure everything is covered with the liquid. Leave to cool until just lukewarm in temperature. Remove the seaweed strips from the bowl of liquid. Add sea salt and hoisin sauce and mix to dissolve the flavorings. Cool completely before using.

TOASTED BROWN RICE

Ingredients:

3 cups	COOKED BROWN RICE	480 g
1 large pc	RED ONION, chopped	120 g
2 cups	MUNG BEAN SPROUTS, root tips removed	60 g
2 tbsp	GREEN ONIONS or GARLIC LEAVES, chopped	7 g
1 pc	NORI SHEET, sushi seaweed, crumbled into tiny bits	4 g
1 tbsp	SUNFLOWER OIL	15 ml
1 tbsp	LIGHT SOY SAUCE	15 ml

RECIPES AND COOKING NOTES

½ tsp	SESAME OIL	15 ml
1 cup	GREEN PEAS, pre-cooked	150 g
1 large pc	CARROT, diced	120 g

(Serves 3)

Procedures:

1. In a large non-stick wok, heat the oil to medium and sauté the onions.
2. Drain the onions in a wire sieve of oil and pat dry with paper towels. Set aside.
3. Using the same wok used in frying the onions, increase heat to high and toast the brown rice quickly, making sure all sides of the grains touch the hot surface of the wok.
4. Add the carrots and green peas and nori pieces and continue stirring the mixture for two minutes.
5. Add the cooked onions, mung bean sprouts, chopped green leaves, sesame oil and soy sauce and cook for a further two minutes before turning off the heat.

USING FROZEN GREEN PEAS

Although lightly boiled to remove enzymes that hasten spoiling, frozen green peas are best precooked before being used with other plant ingredients in a recipe.

Prior cooking for the recipes described here may be done simply by either steaming or lightly boiling.

To eliminate the acrid aftertaste, they may be boiled in slightly salted water for a few minutes.

SUSTAINING A PLANT-BASED DIET WITH FILIPINO FOOD

STAPLE BOWL

Ingredients:

2 cups	COOKED BROWN RICE	320 g
1 cup	COOKED QUINOA	145 g
1 cup	COOKED CORN KERNELS	170 g
1 cup	COOKED RED KIDNEY BEANS or COOKED BROWN LENTILS	180 g
2 tbsp	SESAME SEEDS, toasted	30 g
2 tbsp	TAPIOCA STARCH	16 g
2 tbsp	WATER	30 ml
½ tbsp	ONION FLAKES	5 g
½ tbsp	GARLIC GRANULES	5 g
Dash of	SALT	
1 cup	FIRM TOFU, cut into ¾-inch cubes	240 g
1 tbsp	MAPLE SYRUP	7.5 g
2 tbsp	DIJON MUSTARD	15 g
2 pc	BABY BOK CHOY or *pétsay*, stems discarded, leaves finely chopped	130 g

(Serves 6)

Procedures:

1. Heat and lightly spray a non-stick wok with olive oil to high heat.
2. Put in the brown rice, onion flakes, garlic granules and salt and mix continuously.
3. Add in the quinoa, corn kernels, red kidney beans and the maple syrup-mustard-filled tofu.
4. Continue cooking for three or more minutes, making sure everything is well combined.

RECIPES AND COOKING NOTES

5. Add the chopped bok choy leaves and stir-fry for another minute.

Maple Syrup-Mustard Tofu Cubes

Procedures:

1. For the binder: combine two tablespoons tapioca starch with two tablespoons water to form a paste.
2. For the filling: combine one tablespoon maple syrup with two tablespoons dijon mustard.
3. Make a small cross incision halfway through each tofu cube to make space for filling.
4. Lightly insert maple syrup-mustard mixture into tofu and coat with a little tapioca paste to seal. Roll in sesame seeds.
5. Using an olive oil spray, grease a non-stick wok and set heat to medium.
6. Toast the tofu cubes until lightly browned.

REDUCING THE WATER CONTENT OF FIRM TOFU

The water content of firm tofu is usually reduced before cooking particularly when an outer crisp is desired. This is done by placing kitchen towels or cheesecloth at the bottom of the tofu and weighing it down with a plate for an hour or more before cooking.

Pressing lightly with kitchen towels or even using a salad spinner will work just as fine, in our experience.

The important thing to remember is that the outer part of the tofu is crusted. Lightly trimming this crust before applying pressure to reduce its water content will make the task a little bit easier.

TOFU BISTÉK

Ingredients:

2 blocks	FIRM TOFU, cut into ½-inch thick pieces	900 g
¼ cup	SUNFLOWER OIL, to fry tofu	60 ml
1 large pc	RED ONION, sliced into rings	150 g
2 tbsp	LEMON or *kalamansî* JUICE	30 ml
2 tbsp	SOY SAUCE	30 ml
2 tsp	MAPLE SYRUP	10 ml
2 tbsp	WATER	30 ml
2 tbsp	SUNFLOWER OIL, to sauté	30 ml
To taste,	SALT and PEPPER	

(Serves 3)

Procedures:

1. Cut the tofu in the required size and expel as much water as possible from the tofu pieces by pressing lightly on all sides with kitchen towels.
2. Heat the cooking oil in a non-stick frying pan to medium heat.
3. When the oil is sufficiently hot, reduce heat to low to medium heat and fry the tofu pieces until they form a light golden crust on the skin. Set aside.
4. Heat the oil in a non-stick wok to medium heat.
5. Stir-fry the onion rings just until they change colors and set aside.
6. Add the lemon juice, soy sauce, maple syrup and water and bring to a boil.
7. Season with salt and pepper.
8. When the sauce is reduced and has thickened slightly, add in the fried tofu pieces.

RECIPES AND COOKING NOTES

9. Bring the dish to a boil and turn off the heat. Add the onion rings and serve.

CRISPY FRIED TOFU WITH VINEGAR DIP

Ingredients:

1 block	FIRM TOFU, cut into ¾ inch cubes, fried	400 g
¼ cup	SUNFLOWER OIL	60 ml

(Serves 3)

Procedures:

1. Place the block of tofu in a salad spinner and secure it well by placing cheesecloth on all sides to prevent the tofu from moving while spinning the gadget.
2. Cut the tofu to suggested size.
3. In a non-stick wok, heat the oil to medium heat.
4. Fry the tofu cubes until golden brown and drain well with paper towels.

Vinegar Dip

Ingredients:

¼ cup	BALSAMIC VINEGAR	60 ml
3 tbsp	SOY SAUCE	45 ml
½ pc	RED ONION, chopped	60 g
3 tbsp	COCONUT SUGAR	45 g
Dash of	COARSELY GROUND BLACK PEPPER	

Procedure:

SUSTAINING A PLANT-BASED DIET WITH FILIPINO FOOD

- Mix all the ingredients together, making sure the sugar has completely dissolved before serving.

GREEN BEANS WITH TOFU GISÁDO

Ingredients:

4 cups	GREEN BEANS or ROUND BEANS, sliced thinly	300 g
2 cups	FIRM TOFU, cut into ¾-inch cubes	250 g
4 cloves	GARLIC, minced	16 g
1 pc	RED ONION, halved lengthways and sliced across thinly	120 g
1 pc	TOMATO, chopped	100 g
½ pc	VEGETABLE STOCK CUBE	5 g
1 cup	WATER	250 ml
¼ cup	SUNFLOWER OIL, halved to fry and to sauté	60 ml
To taste,	SALT and PEPPER	

(Serves 3)

Procedures:

1. In a non-stick frying pan, heat two tablespoons of oil to medium heat and stir-fry the tofu until lightly brown on all sides.
2. Drain the fried tofu cubes of excess oil on kitchen towels.
3. Heat the remaining oil in a non-stick wok to medium heat and sauté the garlic until golden brown in color.
4. Add the onions and cook just until they change colors.
5. Add the tomatoes and cook until soft.
6. Pour in the water with the vegetable broth cube.

RECIPES AND COOKING NOTES

7. Season with salt and pepper and leave the broth to boil for a couple of minutes more.
8. Add the sliced beans, reduce heat to simmer and keep watch as the beans will cook quickly.
9. Add the tofu cubes and cover the wok.
10. Turn off heat just as the liquid begins to boil again.

TOFU PAKSÍW WITH LILY BLOSSOMS

Ingredients:

1 block	FIRM TOFU, cut into ½-inch cubes	450 g
3 tbsp	SUNFLOWER OIL, to fry	45 ml
1 tbsp	SUNFLOWER OIL, to sauté	15 ml
¼ cup	WHITE VINEGAR	60 ml
3 tbsp	SOY SAUCE	45 ml
1½ tbsp	COCONUT SUGAR	18 g
6 cloves	GARLIC, crushed	24 g
½ pc	RED ONION, halved lengthways and sliced across thinly	75 g
1 pc	BAY LEAF	
1 cup	DRIED LILY BLOSSOMS	30 g
½ cup	WATER	125 ml

(Serves 3)

Procedures:

1. Cut the tofu to specified size.
2. In a non-stick frying pan, heat the oil to medium heat and fry all sides of the tofu until golden brown in color.
3. Drain the fried tofu of excess oil and set aside.
4. In a non-stick wok, heat the oil to medium heat and brown the garlic.
5. Add the onions and cook just until they change colors.

SUSTAINING A PLANT-BASED DIET WITH FILIPINO FOOD

6. Pour in the vinegar and stir for about a minute before adding the soy sauce, water and sugar.
7. Simmer for ten minutes or more until the sauce is reduced.
8. Add the lily blossoms and cook for five minutes.
9. Add the fried tofu, cover the lid and turn off the heat.

BOK CHOY AND TOFU GISÁDO

Ingredients:

1 block	FIRM TOFU, cut into 1-inch cubes	200 g
2 pc	TOMATOES, chopped	80 g
2 tbsp	WATER	30 ml
4 cloves	GARLIC, minced	16 g
1 pc	RED ONION, halved lengthways and sliced across thinly	70 g
2 tbsp	VEGETARIAN STIR-FRY SAUCE	30 g
¼ cup	SUNFLOWER OIL, to fry	60 g
1 tbsp	SUNFLOWER OIL, to sauté	15 ml
4 pc	BOK CHOY, leaves separated	150 g

(Serves 3)

Procedures:

1. Heat a non-stick frying pan to medium heat and fry the tofu cubes. Drain on paper towels.
2. Heat the oil in a non-stick wok to medium heat.
3. Sauté the garlic until golden brown in color.
4. Add the onions and cook just until they change colors.
5. Add the tomatoes and cook until soft.
6. Pour in the stir-fry sauce and water.

RECIPES AND COOKING NOTES

7. When the sauce gets heated, add in the tofu and bok choy. Cover the lid for one minute and turn off the heat.

TOFU WITH GARLIC LEAVES GISÁDO

Ingredients:

2 cups	GARLIC LEAVES, cut into 2-inch pieces	60 g
2 cups	FIRM TOFU, cut into ¾-inch cubes and fried	300 g
4 cloves	GARLIC, minced	16 g
1½ tbsp	SUNFLOWER OIL	20 ml
2 tbsp	VEGETARIAN STIR-FRY SAUCE	30 ml

(Serves 3)

Procedures:

1. Heat the oil in a wok to medium heat.
2. Add the garlic and sauté until lightly golden brown in color.
3. Add the tofu and garlic leaves and stir fry from seven to ten minutes or until garlic leaves are soft.
4. Stir in the sauce, making sure everything is well coated before turning off the heat.
5. Leave in the heat source until ready to serve.

SUSTAINING A PLANT-BASED DIET WITH FILIPINO FOOD

USING BANANA LEAVES FOR PARCEL COOKING

Cooking by wrapping in banana leaves has traditionally been used for presentation, convenience and the infusion of a unique exotic flavor from the banana leaf that is retained in the food that has been cooked in the parcel.

To heat the banana leaves prior to wrapping, one may use a large enough oven toaster that can accommodate the banana leaves to be used. Preheat the oven toaster, place a banana leaf inside and close the oven toaster cover. You may then monitor readiness of the leaves through the glass cover of the oven toaster.

SPICY TOFU PINÁIS

Ingredients:

1 pack	SILKEN TOFU	300 g
1 tsp	LEMON GRASS STALK, chopped finely	5 g
3 pc	SERRANO PEPPERS, chopped finely	2 g
¼ tsp	FINE TABLE SALT	2 g
½ tsp	COCONUT SUGAR	3 g
	BANANA LEAVES	
	TIE STRINGS	

(Serves 2)

Procedures:

52

RECIPES AND COOKING NOTES

1. Combine the chopped lemon grass stalk, peppers, table salt and coconut sugar together in a bowl and set aside.
2. Wipe the banana leaves with a clean cloth and run through an open fire to make the leaves pliant and soft prior to wrapping.
3. Make well-spaced incisions on top, running lengthwise but not all the way through the bottom of the tofu.
4. Lightly insert the flavorings.
5. Cover with banana leaves, as if wrapping a sandwich and tie with a food-grade string. Do not use plastic or synthetic strings.
6. Heat enough water in an appropriately sized steamer to high heat.
7. When the water reaches a rolling boil, reduce heat to medium and steam the banana wrapped tofu for fifteen minutes.
8. Take out of the steamer and cool slightly before serving with rice.

BITTER GOURD WITH BLACK BEANS GISÁDO

Ingredients:

1 pc	BITTER GOURD or *ampalayá*, halved lengthways and sliced thinly	180 g
3 cloves	GARLIC, minced	12 g
1 can	BLACK BEANS, rinsed in running water and drained	400 g
3 tbsp	VEGETARIAN OYSTER MUSHROOM SAUCE	45 ml
½ pc	VEGETABLE STOCK CUBE	5 g
¼ cup	WATER	60 ml

SUSTAINING A PLANT-BASED DIET WITH FILIPINO FOOD

2 tbsp	SUNFLOWER OIL	30 g
To taste,	SALT and PEPPER	
1 pc	RED ONION, halved lengthways and sliced thinly across	120 g

(Serves 2)

Procedures:

1. Heat the oil in a wok to medium heat and sauté the garlic until golden brown in color.
2. Add the onions and cook just until they change colors.
3. Add the bitter gourd slices and stir-fry for two minutes.
4. Pour in the water and vegetable stock cube.
5. When the liquid begins to boil again, add the black beans.
6. Cook for a further five minutes before adding the vegetarian oyster sauce.
7. Stir-fry for another two minutes to reduce the sauce then turn off the heat.
8. Let the dish sit in the wok over the heat source until ready to serve.

KALE CHIPS

Kale chips are a good snack alternative for when you crave a light in-between meal munch with a crunch.

Ingredients:

1 bunch	KALE, leaves separated	500 g
1 tbsp	SUNFLOWER OIL	15 ml
1 tsp	FINE TABLE SALT	5 g

(Serves 2)

RECIPES AND COOKING NOTES

Procedures:

1. Wash the kale with water and dry in a salad spinner.
2. Tear the leaves into 2-inch pieces and discard the hard stems.
3. Arrange in a baking paper-lined sheet and rub each piece with oil and salt.
4. Bake in a preheated 180°C oven for fifteen minutes but watch the oven while cooking and remove the ones that are already done.
5. When all of the kale leaves have been cooked, take out the baking sheet and let the kale rest for five more minutes in the hot sheet before cooling.

KALE AND WHITE BEAN DIP

Ingredients:

1 can	CANNELLINI BEANS, drained	400 g
2 cups	KALE LEAVES	110 g
2 cloves	GARLIC	8 g
1 tbsp	OLIVE OIL	15 ml
2 tbsp	LEMON JUICE	30 ml
3 tbsp	UNSALTED CASHEW NUTS, soaked overnight	15 g
1 tbsp	MAPLE SYRUP	15 ml

Procedures:

- Put all ingredients together in a blender and pulse until smooth. Store in an airtight container in the refrigerator until needed.

BINDING MINCED INGREDIENTS WITHOUT EGGS

1. OKRA-WATER BINDER

Ingredients:

10 pc	OKRA LADY FINGER, sliced thinly	100 g
¾ cup	WATER	180 ml

Procedure:

In a small pot, place the water with the sliced okra and bring to a boil to high heat. When the water reaches a rolling boil, reduce heat to low and simmer for twenty minutes. Discard the pulp by passing though a sieve. Cool completely before using.

2. TARO-WATER BINDER

Ingredients:

1 large pc	TARO, quartered	200 g
4 cups	WATER	1 L

Procedure:

Place the taro and water in a cooking pot and bring to a boil to high heat. When the water reaches a rolling boil, reduce heat to medium-to-low and cook covered for 35 minutes. Lift the lid and continue cooking for 15 minutes more to reduce the liquid. Remove the cooked taro and save the water. Cool completely before using.

RECIPES AND COOKING NOTES

TOFU-TARO SIOMAI

Ingredients:

1 block	FIRM TOFU	250 g
1 cup	TARO, cooked and mashed	180 g
½ can	WATER CHESTNUTS, drained and chopped finely	60 g
1 small pc	CARROT, finely chopped	100 g
3 stalks	GREEN ONIONS, finely chopped	20 g
1 large pc	RED ONIONS, finely chopped	180 g
1 pc	VEGETABLE STOCK CUBE, chicken-style, crushed	10 g
½ tsp	FINE TABLE SALT	2.5 g
1 tbsp	LIGHT SOY SAUCE	15 ml
2 tsp	SESAME OIL	10 ml
½ tsp	CHINESE FIVE-SPICE POWDER	2.5 g
3 tbsp	OKRA-WATER or TARO-WATER	45 ml
40 pc	SHANGHAI WONTON SKIN	270 g

(Serves 5)

Procedures:

1. Leave the tofu overnight in the freezer.
2. Thaw the tofu until completely soft.
3. Cut the tofu into small pieces that you can handle.
4. Expel as much water as possible from the thawed tofu pieces by manually pressing on each piece.
5. Shred the tofu in mince pieces into a mixing bowl.
6. Add the taro and mix until it gels into one sticky mass.
7. Add crushed vegetable stock cube, salt, light soy sauce, sesame oil and five-spice powder and blend well.
8. Add the water chestnuts, carrots, green onions, and onions and mix thoroughly.

SUSTAINING A PLANT-BASED DIET WITH FILIPINO FOOD

9. Add the okra water and mix with a rubber scraper until the water has been absorbed by the mixture.
10. Place wonton wrapper in the middle of palm as thumb and index finger slightly touch.
11. Form a depression by pressing in the middle of the wonton skin.
12. Place a tablespoon of the siomai mixture in the center and seal the sides while leaving the top uncovered.
13. Repeat until all of the mixture has been used up.
14. Place enough water in the steamer boiler of a large steamer and bring to a boil to high heat.
15. When the water reaches a rolling boil, reduce heat to medium and prepare the steamer cooker.
16. Arrange the siomai in the steamer cooker, making sure there is enough space among them so steam can pass through and cook each one evenly.
17. Steam for 20–25 minutes.
18. Move the cooked siomai in a platter that has been lined with non-stick baking paper.
19. Cool slightly and serve with balsamic vinegar-light soy sauce dip.

Balsamic Vinegar-Light Soy Sauce Dip

Ingredients:

¾ cup	BALSAMIC VINEGAR	180 ml
½ cup	LIGHT SOY SAUCE	125 ml
3 cloves	GARLIC, minced	12 g
2 tsp	GINGER, slice into small sticks	10 g
1 tsp	SESAME OIL	5 ml
2 tsp	MAPLE SYRUP	10 ml

Procedure:

-   Mix all ingredients together and serve with the tofu-taro siomai.

RECIPES AND COOKING NOTES

USING TEXTURED VEGETABLE PROTEIN (TVP)

Also known as textured soy protein, the product was popularized in the Philippines during the martial law years as a meat alternative. Since then, it has been widely-used as meat extender owing to the product's capability to absorb the flavors of the dishes it augments.

Textured vegetable protein is a by-product of extracting oil from soybeans which are then cooked and desiccated into mince-sized pieces. Hence, it is marketed as a defatted soy product.

Being a processed food ingredient, stricter adherents of plant-based eating may have issues about its use. It has been added in this collection with a few popular recipes to demonstrate its efficient flavor-absorbing capability in the food that we love.

Between a choice of meat, poultry, seafood and dairy, it is easy to opt for TVP. However, fresh plant-based ingredients should take precedence over processed products as a rule.

TÁPA BITS TOPPINGS

Ingredients:

1 cup, dry	TEXTURED VEGETABLE PROTEIN	85 g
½ cup	HOT WATER	125 ml
½ tsp	VEGETABLE STOCK CUBE, beef style	5 g
¼ cup	WHITE VINEGAR	60 ml
1 tsp	SEA SALT	5 ml

SUSTAINING A PLANT-BASED DIET WITH FILIPINO FOOD

8 cloves	GARLIC, minced	32 g
1½ tbsp	COCONUT SUGAR	11 g
Dash of	GROUND BLACK PEPPER	
1 tbsp	SUNFLOWER OIL, to marinate	15 ml
2 tbsp	SUNFLOWER OIL, to stir-fry	30 ml
2 cloves	GARLIC, to stir-fry	8 g

(Serves 3)

Procedures:

1. Pass the textured vegetable protein through a wire mesh sieve to remove the powdered parts.
2. Sort out and select one cup from the bigger bits to use in the recipe. Set aside.
3. In a non-stick frying pan, heat a tablespoon of sunflower oil to medium heat and fry the garlic until golden brown in color. Cool slightly.
4. In a small pot, dissolve the vegetable stock cube in hot water.
5. Add the fried garlic with the oil, vinegar, salt, coconut sugar, black pepper.
6. Bring to a boil to medium heat and reduce heat to simmer when it begins to boil.
7. Let the liquid cook for ten minutes to combine flavors as well as to reduce the acidity of the vinegar.
8. Turn off heat and add the textured vegetable protein.
9. Transfer to a porcelain bowl and cool completely after which rest the mixture in the refrigerator for at least two hours before cooking.
10. Heat the oil in a non-stick wok to medium heat and sauté the garlic until golden brown in color.
11. Add the marinated textured vegetable protein.
12. Stir-fry continuously until all liquid has dried up and the textured vegetable protein has started to firm up but being careful as well not to overcook.
13. Transfer into a serving bowl and cool slightly before serving as a topping to your choice of rice.

RECIPES AND COOKING NOTES

MEATLESS LÓNGGANÍSA

Ingredients:

1 cup, dry	TEXTURED VEGETABLE PROTEIN	85 g
¾ cup	HOT WATER	180 ml
2 tbsp	FLAXSEED MEAL	16 g
1 tbsp	TAPIOCA STARCH	8 g
½ pc	VEGETABLE STOCK CUBE	5 g
8 cloves	GARLIC, minced	32 g
2 tsp	SOY SAUCE	10 ml
1 tsp	WHITE VINEGAR	5 ml
To taste,	SALT	
To taste,	GROUND BLACK PEPPER	
3 tbsp	COCONUT SUGAR	45 g
12 pc	PLASTIC WRAPPER, 5-inch squares	120 g

(Serves 5)

Procedures:

1. In a separate cup dissolve the flaxseed or linseed meal in two tablespoons hot water and set aside.
2. Add a tablespoon of water and dissolve the tapioca starch in another container.
3. Combine the two preceding mixtures together with the crushed vegetable stock cube with the hot water in a 500–ml liquid measuring cup and mix well.
4. Rest the mixture for at least an hour.
5. When the mixture is fully rested and cooled and all the liquid is fully absorbed by the dry ingredients, transfer the mixture to a larger mixing bowl.
6. Add the garlic, white vinegar, salt, black pepper and sugar in the same cup and mix well.

SUSTAINING A PLANT-BASED DIET WITH FILIPINO FOOD

7. Rest the mixture for another hour, covered with a plastic wrap in the refrigerator.
8. Wrap into small 30-gram pieces and pack in a well sealed freezer bag and store in the freezer until required.

PICADILLO WITH SWEET POTATOES AND SABÁ

Ingredients:

1 cup, dry	TEXTURED VEGETABLE PROTEIN	85 g
14 tbsp	BOILING WATER	218 ml
2½ tsp	CALDERETA MIX	12 g
Dash of	SALT and PEPPER	
2 tbsp	SUNFLOWER OIL	30 ml
1 large pc	RED ONION, chopped	120 g
4 cloves	GARLIC, minced	16 g
To taste,	FISH SAUCE SUBSTITUTE, recipe on p. 43	
1can	DICED ITALIAN TOMATOES	400 g
½ pc	VEGETABLE STOCK CUBE	5 g
½ cup	HOT WATER	125 ml
2 pc	SWEET POTATOES, diced	220 g
3 pc	PLANTAIN BANANAS or *sabá*, diced	240 g
large pc	CARROT, diced	120 g
3 tbsp	DRIED CRANBERRIES or RAISINS	40 g

(Serves 4)

Procedures:

1. Heat the oil in a large non-stick wok to medium heat.
2. Add garlic and sauté until golden brown in color.

RECIPES AND COOKING NOTES

3. Add the onions and cook just until they change colors.
4. Add the textured vegetable protein and stir-fry for three minutes.
5. Pour in the tomatoes and vegetable broth and simmer until the sauce is slightly reduced, or about seven minutes.
6. Season with the fish oil substitute and add the sweet potatoes, plantains and carrots.
7. Cook for another three minutes.
8. When the liquid has turned into a thick sauce, the dish is ready for serving.

STIR-FRIED MIXED VEGETABLES

Ingredients:

1 large pc	BROCCOLI, florets separated	380 g
1 large pc	CARROT, sliced diagonally with slices cut in half after	140 g
1 cup	SNOW PEAS, stringed	130 g
8–10 pc	BABY CORN	60 g
1 small pc	CAULIFLOWER, florets separated	350 g
3 stalks	CELERY, cut into ½-in long pieces	210 g
1 large pc	CHINESE CABBAGE or *wombok*, cut into ½-inch across the leaves and stems	370 g
4 cloves	GARLIC, minced	16 g
1 tbsp	GINGER, julienned	40 g
2 tbsp	SUNFLOWER OIL	30 ml
3 tbsp	VEGETARIAN STIR-FRY SAUCE	45 ml
To taste,	SALT	
1 large pc	RED ONION, halved and sliced thinly	140 g

(Serves 4)

63

SUSTAINING A PLANT-BASED DIET WITH FILIPINO FOOD

Procedures:

1. In a large stockpot, add enough water to cover all the prepared vegetables and add a tablespoon of salt.
2. Set heat to high and bring to a boil.
3. When the water reaches a rolling boil, reduce heat to simmer and add the vegetables, except the cabbage.
4. After thirty seconds, add the cabbage.
5. Wait for another thirty seconds to drain the liquid from the blanched vegetables in a large sieve or strainer.
6. Pass through running water to stop vegetables from cooking.
7. Drain well.
8. In a large non-stick wok, heat the sunflower oil to high.
9. Add the garlic and sauté until golden brown in color.
10. Add the onions and ginger and stir-fry until soft and fragrant.
11. Add the stir-fry sauce until well heated.
12. Add the vegetables all at once and mix well. Turn off the heat.
13. Continue stirring until everything is coated with the sauce.

RECIPES AND COOKING NOTES

BLANCHING VEGETABLES IN SALTED WATER

Blanching vegetables in salted water before a stir-fry is an excellent way to prepare fresh vegetables. A little bit of salt is added in blanching water to eliminate the mild acrid taste that comes from the sap of some vegetables.

Once mixed vegetables are blanched with salted water, the function of the stir-fry will only be limited to augmenting flavors from sauté vegetables and the stir-fry sauce.

Because of the efficiently-timed blanch and the overall decreased time required for cooking, vegetables are sure to have a crispy texture even after being cooked in oil.

LUMPIYÂ PLATE

Ingredients:

1 pc	CARROT, pared, peeled and julienned	90 g
1 pc	SWEET POTATO, peeled and julienned	120 g
1 pc	JICAMA or *singkamás*, peeled and julienned	100 g
2 stalks	CELERY, sliced thinly	120 g
¼ pc	CABBAGE, sliced thinly	300 g
5 pc	ROUND BEANS, sliced thinly	50 g
1 can	CHICKPEAS, washed and drained	400 g
4 cups	WATER	1 L
2 pc	VEGETABLE STOCK CUBES, chicken-style	20 g
To taste,	SALT and PEPPER	

SUSTAINING A PLANT-BASED DIET WITH FILIPINO FOOD

| 1 pc | RED ONION, halved lengthways and sliced across thinly | 120 g |

(Serves 5)

Procedures:

1. Combine water, onion, vegetable stock cubes, salt and pepper in a large enough cooking pot to medium-high heat. Bring to a boil.
2. When the pot reaches a rolling boil, leave the liquid boiling briskly for five more minutes to let the flavors combine thoroughly.
3. Reduce heat to simmer. Drop in the chickpeas, cabbage, green beans and sweet potatoes.
4. After thirty seconds, add the carrots and celery and cook for a further minute and a half.
5. Turn off heat and drain in a pasta strainer or sieve.
6. Transfer to a serving plate when slightly cooled.

Lumpiyâ Sauce

Ingredients:

½ cup	COCONUT SUGAR	100 g
2 tbsp	SOY SAUCE	30 ml
2 cups	WATER, for the sauce	500 ml
¼ cup	TAPIOCA STARCH	40 g
¼ cup	WATER, as thickener	60 ml
¼ cup	TOASTED PEANUTS, crushed	40 g
2 tbsp	FRIED GARLIC, crushed	30 g

Procedures:

1. Combine tapioca starch with water. Mix well and set aside.
2. In a small pan, melt half of the sugar to medium heat.

RECIPES AND COOKING NOTES

3. When the sugar thickens and turns golden brown, pour in water, soy sauce and the remaining sugar.
4. Continue cooking and wait until everything is well combined and the sauce is slightly reduced.
5. Add the tapioca starch and mix thoroughly.
6. Reduce heat and cook until the sauce is thick enough to pour.
7. Serve the sauce with the vegetables and top with fried garlic and toasted peanuts.

LUMPIYÂNG PRÍTO

Ingredients:

20 pc	SMALL LUMPIYÂ WRAPPERS,	
	5-inch x 5-inch squares	250 g
1 cup	WATER, to seal edges	250 ml
½ cup	SUNFLOWER OIL	125 ml
1 mixing	LUMPIYÂ PLATE, recipe on p. 66	

(Serves 3)

Procedures:

1. Lay the wrapper, opposite pointed edges vertically aligned with you.
2. Place two tablespoonfuls of the lumpiyâ plate mixture near the center and fold the edges inward.
3. Brush the top edge of the wrapper with water and lift the lower edge near the center.
4. Fold downside upwards until it seals at the point where you brushed the top edge of the wrapper with water.
5. Heat the oil in a non-stick wok to low–medium heat.
6. Fry the lumpiyâ until golden brown in color.
7. Drain on kitchen towels to remove excess oil.

SUSTAINING A PLANT-BASED DIET WITH FILIPINO FOOD

8. Serve with vinegar dip.

Lumpiyâ Dip

Ingredients:

2 cloves	GARLIC, minced	8 g
¼ cup	BALSAMIC VINEGAR	60 ml
3 tbsp	LIGHT SOY SAUCE	45 g
Dash of	COARSELY GROUND BLACK PEPPER	

Procedure:

- Mix all ingredients together and serve with the lumpi-yâng príto.

MANGO CUCUMBER ENSALÁDA

Ingredients:

2 pc	GREEN MANGOES, pitted and diced small	240 g
1 cup, dry	BULGUR WHEAT	250 g
	BOILING WATER, to cover wheat	
1 large pc	RED ONION, chopped	180 g
1 pc	LEBANESE CUCUMBER, halved, deseeded and diced	120 g
2 cups	FRESH FLAT-LEAF PARSLEY, chopped	180 g
1 cup	BABY SPINACH LEAVES, chopped	70 g
¼ cup	FRESH MINT, chopped	30 g
¼ cup	VEGETABLE BROTH	60 ml
1 pc	LEMON	50 g
To taste,	SALT and PEPPER	

RECIPES AND COOKING NOTES

(Serves 3)

Procedures:

1. Put the bulgur wheat in a ceramic bowl and cover with enough boiling water.
2. Let the wheat soak in the water until cool for at least an hour.
3. Transfer to a large mixing bowl and add all the dry ingredients in and mix well.
4. Drizzle the vegetable broth while mixing to let the salad ingredients absorb the broth.
5. Juice the lemons and repeat mixing of ingredients as with the vegetable broth.
6. Check the seasonings and correct as necessary.
7. Cover with cling wrap and rest in the refrigerator for half an hour before serving.

KALE QUINOA ENSALADÁ

Ingredients:

1 bunch	KALE, leaves separated, hard stems discarded	500 g
2 cups	COOKED QUINOA	290 g
½ cup	PEPITAS or squash seeds	125 g
½ cup	DRIED CRANBERRIES	90 g
½ tbsp	OLIVE OIL	8 g
1 tbsp	MAPLE SYRUP	15 ml
3 tbsp	BALSAMIC VINEGAR	45 ml

(Serves 4)

Procedures:

SUSTAINING A PLANT-BASED DIET WITH FILIPINO FOOD

1. Mix the balsamic vinegar, maple syrup and the olive oil together in a small bowl.
2. Chop the kale leaves into fine pieces and mix together with the cooked quinoa, pepitas and dried cranberries.
3. Drizzle the vinegar mixture a little at a time on the salad mixture while continuously mixing with a large spoon.
4. Transfer into a covered container and chill in the refrigerator for at least an hour before serving.

ÓKOY

Ingredients:

½ cup	WHOLEMEAL FLOUR	60 g
½ cup	OAT FLOUR	55 g
2 large pc	SWEET POTATOES, grated into long thin strands	520 g
1 large pc	CARROT, grated into long thin strands	180
2 cups	MUNG BEAN SPROUTS, tips removed	250 g
1 large pc	RED ONION, finely chopped	120 g
3 stalks	GREEN ONIONS, chopped	20 g
1 pack	TOFU, cut into ½-in x ½-in x ¼-in pieces	250 g
1 pc	VEGETABLE STOCK CUBE, crushed	10 g
Dash of	COARSELY GROUND BLACK PEPPER	
To taste	SEA SALT	
1 tbsp	FLAXSEED MEAL	15 g
1 cup	ICE COLD WATER	250 ml
1 cup	SUNFLOWER OIL, to fry	250 ml

(Serves 5)

Procedures:

RECIPES AND COOKING NOTES

1. Put half a cup of rolled oats in a blender and pulse until the oats turn into powder.
2. Transfer to a mixing bowl and add the whole-meal flour, vegetable stock cube, flaxseed meal and sea salt and mix well.
3. Stir in the water and mix until there are no visible lumps.
4. Add in the vegetables and the tofu and mix well.
5. Heat the oil in a non-stick wok to medium heat and fry the batter in single batches of a fourth of a cup each until done.
6. Drain in a sieve or colander before transferring to a platter that is lined with kitchen towels.

Garlic Vinegar Dip

Ingredients:

½ cup	COCONUT VINEGAR	125 ml
4 cloves	GARLIC, minced	16 g
Dash of	COARSELY GROUND BLACK PEPPER	
To taste	SEA SALT	
2 pc	SERRANO PEPPERS, chopped (optional)	2 g

Procedures:

- Mix all ingredients together and serve with the fried ókoy.

SUSTAINING A PLANT-BASED DIET WITH FILIPINO FOOD

SUBSTITUTING VINEGARS FOR VARIETY

Coconut vinegar has been a traditional Filipino cooking ingredient. Its different uses include being a flavoring ingredient, a preservative, a souring agent to quasi-cook our raw meat and raw seafood delicacies and as a dipping sauce liquid base.

By using vinegars and condiments that are not native to us, however, we can attain a variety of flavors to augment the taste foundation that has been substantially diminished with the exclusion of meat, seafood and dairy in our cooking.

As a vinegar dip, try using balsamic vinegar with light soy sauce instead of the traditional salt or dark soy sauce.

PINAKBÉT

This recipe is a variation of the traditional Ilocano way of cooking the dish by braising or kúlob, in Filipino, with liquid bagoóng as both a liquid base as well as salty flavoring ingredient.

Ingredients:

4 pc	EGGPLANTS, cut into 1-inch long pieces	400 g
1 pc small	BITTER GOURD, halved, seeds removed, and sliced thinly	200 g
10 pc	ÓKRA LADY FINGER	100 g
1 bundle	SNAKE BEANS, cut into 2-inch long pieces	300 g
2 pc	SWEET POTATOES, peeled and cut into 1-inch cubes	200 g
3 pc	TARO or *gábe*, peeled and cut into 1-inch cubes	240 g

RECIPES AND COOKING NOTES

3 pc	GREEN CHILLI PEPPERS	60 g
½ pc small	SQUASH or PUMPKIN, cut into 1-inch cubes	520 g
50 pc	LIMA BEANS, partially cooked	65 g
1 pc	VEGETABLE STOCK CUBE, chicken-style	20 g
1 pc.	RED ONION, halved lengthways and sliced across thinly	100 g
5 cloves	GARLIC, minced	20 g
2 large pc	TOMATO, chopped	60 g
1 cup	WATER	250 ml
1 tbsp	LIGHT SOY SAUCE	30 g
1 tbsp	GINGER, crushed	30 g

(Serves 4)

Procedures:

1. To prepare the lima beans, soak a cup of beans in filtered water overnight.
2. In a wire sieve, rinse in running water and discard the unusable pieces.
3. Heat a liter of water in a cooking pot to medium heat.
4. When the water reaches a rolling boil, reduce heat to low-to-medium heat and drop in the lima beans.
5. After forty minutes of cooking, select from the cooking pot the required amount of lima beans and continue cooking the rest for another forty minutes or until done.
6. In a large cooking pot, mix water, vegetable stock cube, onions, tomatoes and crushed ginger.
7. Bring to a boil to high heat.
8. When the water reaches a rolling boil, reduce heat to simmer and add the light soy sauce.
9. Arrange the vegetables in the pot in this order from the bottom: taro, sweet potatoes, squash, snake beans, lima beans, bitter gourd, ókra, green chilli peppers and egg-plants.

SUSTAINING A PLANT-BASED DIET WITH FILIPINO FOOD

10. Cook for five minutes.
11. Without removing the cover, turn the vegetables over by holding the handles with hands on potholders and tossing the contents.
12. Repeat this for three to four times until you are sure the vegetables have all been turned.
13. Cook for another ten minutes and check, return to heat and repeat procedure until all vegetables are properly cooked.
14. Serve with rice.

STIR-FRIED PINAKBÉT VEGETABLES

This recipe is a stir-fry that uses the same vegetables used in pinakbét.

Ingredients:

4 pc	EGGPLANTS, cut into 1-inch thick pieces	400 g
1 pc small	BITTER GOURD, halved, seeds removed, and sliced thinly	200 g
10 pc	ÓKRA LADY FINGER	100 g
1 bundle	SNAKE BEANS, cut into 2-inch long pieces	300 g
3 pc	GREEN CHILLI PEPPERS	60 g
2 pc	SWEET POTATOES, peeled and cut into 1-inch cubes	200 g
3 pc	TARO or *gábe*, peeled and cut into 1-inch cubes	240 g
½ pc	SQUASH or PUMPKIN, cut into 1-inch cubes	520 g
2 tsp	SALT, to blanch	10 g
1 pc	VEGETABLE STOCK CUBE	20 g
4 cups	WATER, to steam	1 L

RECIPES AND COOKING NOTES

2 tbsp	SUNFLOWER OIL	30 ml
1 pc	RED ONION, halved lengthways and sliced thinly across	100 g
5 cloves	GARLIC, minced	20 g
1 large pc	TOMATO, chopped	20 g
¼ cup	WATER, to cook	60 ml
¼ cup	VEGETARIAN STIR-FRY SAUCE	60 ml

(Serves 5)

Procedures:

1. Place enough water in a steamer boiler to cook all the vegetables in this recipe. Add in salt and the vegetable stock cube.
2. Bring to a boil to high heat.
3. When the water reaches a rolling boil, reduce heat to medium and prepare the steamer cooker.
4. Arrange the vegetables in such a way that you can take out the ones to cook first with ease.
5. The following is the approximate cooking times for the pinakbét vegetables: sweet potatoes and taro will cook in twenty minutes, squash or pumpkin in fifteen minutes, snake beans and eggplants in ten minutes and bitter gourd, okra and green chillies in five minutes.
6. Combine everything in a mixing bowl and prepare to sauté immediately.
7. In a non-stick wok, heat the oil to medium and sauté the garlic until golden brown in color.
8. Add the onions and cook just until they change colors.
9. Add the tomatoes and cook until soft.
10. Pour in the vegetarian stir-fry sauce and the water and bring to a boil.
11. Cook until the sauce is slightly reduced and thickened or about five minutes.
12. Add the vegetables and stir-fry until everything is well combined.
13. Transfer to a serving platter and serve.

SUSTAINING A PLANT-BASED DIET WITH FILIPINO FOOD

SÓTANGHÓN GISÁDO

This vermicelli dish is a variation of the traditional recipe of Pansít Gisádo which is usually based on the rice noodle called bíhon in Filipino.

Ingredients:

1 pack	VERMICELLI BEAN THREADS	250 g
1 pc	CARROT, julienned	120 g
¼ pc	CABBAGE, sliced thinly	300 g
2 stalks	CELERY, sliced thinly	120 g
10 pc	ROUND BEANS, stringed and cut into 2-inch lengths	100 g
½ cup, dry	BLACK FUNGUS or *taingáng dagâ*, rehydrated	40 g
2 tbsp	SUNFLOWER OIL	30 ml
4 cloves	GARLIC, minced	16 g
1 pc	VEGETABLE STOCK CUBES, chicken-style, dissolved in	10 g
1½ cups	HOT WATER	175 ml
3 tbsp	SOY SAUCE	45 ml
2 tbsp	VEGETARIAN STIR-FRY SAUCE	30 ml
Dash of	COARSELY GROUND BLACK PEPPER	
1 large pc	RED ONION, halved lengthways and sliced thinly across	120 g

(Serves 4)

Procedures:

1. In a mixing bowl, soften the mung bean threads in cold water, drain and set aside.
2. Heat the oil in a non-stick wok to medium heat.
3. Add the garlic and sauté until golden brown in color.

RECIPES AND COOKING NOTES

4. Stir in the onions and cook just until they change colors.
5. Add the black fungus and stir-fry for another minute.
6. Add the vegetable stock and bring to a boil.
7. Season with soy sauce and vegetarian stir-fry sauce.
8. When the liquid gets boiling again, add the sliced cabbage and cover to soften.
9. Add the beans, celery and carrots and simmer without cover for two to three minutes.
10. Increase heat to high and add the mung bean threads and continue mixing until all the liquid has been absorbed.

USING SÓTANGHÓN OR GLASS NOODLES

Also known as cellophane noodles or glass noodles because of the crystal-clear strands, vermicelli bean threads are made from mung bean starch.

Consistently certified as a food item with a low glycemic index, vermicelli are in the same class as the darker-colored sweet potato noodles famously known in Korean cooking.

Vermicelli may also be used as a filler for lumpiyâ recipes, steamed dumplings and cooked to augment a Vietnamese-style salad wrap.

SÓTANGHÓN WITH BOTTLE GOURD

Ingredients:

4 cups	BOTTLE GOURD or *upô*, diced	650 g
1 pack	VERMICELLI BEAN THREADS	100 g
2 tbsp	SUNFLOWER OIL	30 ml

SUSTAINING A PLANT-BASED DIET WITH FILIPINO FOOD

4 cloves	GARLIC, minced	16 g
1 pc	TOMATO, chopped	100 g
1 large pc	RED ONION, halved and sliced thinly	140 g
4 cups	WATER	1 L
2 pc	VEGETABLE STOCK CUBES	20 g
1 tbsp	VEGETARIAN OYSTER MUSHROOM SAUCE	15 ml

(Serves 4)

Procedures:

1. Heat the cooking oil in a non-stick wok to medium heat and sauté the garlic until golden brown in color.
2. Add the onions and cook just until they change colors.
3. Add the tomatoes and cook until soft.
4. Add the bottle gourd and oyster mushroom sauce and stir-fry for a couple of minutes.
5. Pour in the water together with the vegetable stock cubes.
6. Cover and cook for five minutes.
7. Add the vermicelli bean threads and cook without cover until both the bottle gourd and glass noodles are cooked.

LAKSÁ-LAKSÁ

Ingredients:

2 cups	BANANA BLOSSOMS, finely chopped, to clean and prepare banana blossoms please refer to p. 81	170 g
1 cup	SNAKE BEANS, cut into 1-inch long pieces	80 g

RECIPES AND COOKING NOTES

1 cup	EGGPLANT, sliced diagonally	130 g
1 cup	SQUASH or PUMPKIN, cut into	
	1-inch cubes	140 g
2 cups	SQUASH LEAVES AND STEMS	60 g
3 pc	VEGETABLE STOCK CUBES	30 g
3 cups	WATER	750 ml
1 pack	VERMICELLI BEAN THREADS	100 g
2 tbsp	SUNFLOWER OIL	60 ml
4 cloves	GARLIC, minced	16 g
1 large pc	RED ONION, sliced	120 g
To taste,	SALT and PEPPER	

(Serves 4)

Procedures:

1. Heat oil in a large non-stick wok to medium heat and sauté the garlic until golden brown in color.
2. Add the onions and cook just until they change colors.
3. Add the banana blossoms, snake beans, pumpkin and eggplants and stir-fry for a couple of minutes.
4. Pour in the water and the vegetable stock cubes and bring to a boil.
5. Cook until the vegetables are almost ready.
6. Add the noodles and the young squash leaves and stems and season with salt and pepper.
7. Reduce heat and cook until both noodles and vegetables are cooked.

SUSTAINING A PLANT-BASED DIET WITH FILIPINO FOOD

USING AND CLEANING FRESH BANANA BLOSSOMS

Aside from being economical to use, fresh banana blossoms are always preferred over the more convenient choice that we get brined and canned from the supermarket.

To clean fresh banana blossoms, remove and discard the tough outer leaves, chop and set aside in a mixing bowl, add generous amount of salt and a little water to work and mix thoroughly, as if rinsing hand-washed laundry. Take a handful at a time and squeeze out the brine from the banana blossom pieces and set aside in another bowl. When most of the brine has been squeezed out, cover the banana blossom pieces with new water for at least an hour. Expel the water and set aside to cook.

SÓTANGHÓN HOT POT

Ingredients:

4 cups	WATER	1 L
1 large pc	RED ONION, halved lengthways and sliced thinly across	150 g
1 tbsp	GINGER, julienned	20 g
3 stalks	GREEN ONIONS, cut into 2-in long pieces	20 g
1 cup	BUTTON MUSHROOMS, quartered	
1 can	BABY CORN, rinsed and drained	400 g
1 large pc	CARROT, sliced diagonally	120 g
½ pc	CHINESE CABBAGE, hard stems cut-off and leaves sliced	250 g
2 pc	VEGETABLE STOCK CUBES	20 g
1½ tbsp	VEGETARIAN STIR-FRY SAUCE	22 ml

RECIPES AND COOKING NOTES

¼ cup	FRIED GARLIC, to garnish	24 g
½ cup	GREEN ONIONS, finely chopped, to garnish	30 g
1 pack	VERMICELLI BEAN THREADS	100 g

(Serves 4)

Procedures:

1. In a large pot, combine water, vegetable stock cubes, stir-fry sauce, onions, ginger and green onions.
2. Bring to a rolling boil to medium heat.
3. After five minutes of boiling, reduce heat to simmer and add the baby corn, mushrooms and carrots.
4. Cook for another three minutes, when the pot begins to boil again.
5. Add the mung bean threads and the cabbage and cover for three more minutes.
6. Turn off heat and rest for a minute before serving.

SÓTANGHÓN WITH SPONGE GOURD

Ingredients:

4 cups	SPONGE GOURD or *patóla*, diced	600 g
1 pack	VERMICELLI BEAN THREADS	100 g
2 tbsp	SUNFLOWER OIL	30 ml
4 cloves	GARLIC, minced	16 g
1 pc	TOMATO, chopped	100 g
1 large pc	RED ONION, halved lengthways and sliced thinly across	140 g
4 cups	WATER	1 l
2 pc	VEGETABLE STOCK CUBES, chicken-style	20 g
1 tbsp	VEGETARIAN OYSTER MUSHROOM	

SUSTAINING A PLANT-BASED DIET WITH FILIPINO FOOD

SAUCE   15 ml

(Serves 4)

Procedures:

1. Heat the cooking oil in a non-stick wok to medium heat and sauté the garlic until golden brown in color.
2. Add the onions and cook just until they change colors.
3. Add the tomatoes and cook until soft.
4. Add the sponge gourd and oyster mushroom sauce and stir-fry for a couple of minutes.
5. Pour in the water together with the vegetable stock cubes and bring to a boil.
6. Cover and cook for five minutes.
7. Add the vermicelli bean threads and cook uncovered until both the bottle gourd and noodles are cooked.

SÓTANGHÓN ASÁDO NOODLES

The stock of this vermicelli vegetable soup takes after the soup of the familiar beef asádo mámi which is a favorite snack item to warm the stomach. We substituted vermicelli for the traditional egg noodles to make it vegan-friendly.

Ingredients:

1 pack	VERMICELLI BEAN THREADS or *sótanghón*	100 g
4 cloves	GARLIC, crushed whole	16 g
1 pc	BAY LEAF	
2 tsp	GINGER, slivered	15 g
1 pc	STAR ANISE	
1 section	BOTTLE GOURD or *úpo*, peeled, deseeded and diced	400 g

RECIPES AND COOKING NOTES

1 large pc	CARROT, sliced diagonally	120 g
½ pc	CHINESE CABBAGE or *pétsay baguio*, hard stem cut, leaves sliced	250 g
To taste,	SALT and PEPPER	
2 cups	WATER	500 ml
1 pc	VEGETABLE STOCK CUBE, beef-style	10 g
1 tbsp	LIGHT SOY SAUCE	15 g
½ tbsp	COCONUT SUGAR	8 g
¼ cup	FRIED GARLIC, to garnish	24 g
½ cup	GREEN ONIONS, finely chopped, to garnish	30 g
1 pc	RED ONION, quartered	120 g

(Serves 4)

Procedures:

1. Combine water, vegetable stock cube, onion, garlic, bay leaf, ginger and star anise in a pot and bring to a boil to medium heat.
2. Let the soup base boil briskly for ten to fifteen minutes, making sure the liquid isn't reduced too much. Add water as needed. The bay leaf, ginger, star anise and garlic may be removed at this point.
3. Add the vermicelli, bottle gourd and carrots and boil for another five minutes.
4. Add the light soy sauce and sugar and continue boiling for two more minutes.
5. Add the cabbage, turn off heat and cover the pot.
6. Let it rest for three minutes more for the Chinese cabbage to cook.
7. Serve with fried garlic bits and chopped green onions.

SUSTAINING A PLANT-BASED DIET WITH FILIPINO FOOD

USING TRADITIONAL FRUIT VEGETABLES

Our traditional fruit vegetables range from those with distinct tastes such as bitter gourds, peppers and eggplants which approximate a certain meaty taste when broiled to the ones with less imposing tastes like sponge gourds, bottle gourds and the chayote squash.

A number of dishes have been created that highlight the taste of our vegetables with distinct tastes but the latter ones are not really without merit. This is primarily due to their capacity to blend into flavor combination in the dishes they are included in.

They do well also when plainly sautéed in garlic, onions and tomatoes. Instead of using whole eggs to thicken the vege-table broth, try using a chickpea flour thickener.

BANANA BLOSSOMS WITH SÓTANGHÓN

Ingredients:

1 pc	BANANA BLOSSOM, cleaned and chopped, please see p. 81	350 g
1 pack	VERMICELLI BEAN THREADS	100 g
4 cups	WATER	1 L
2 tbsp	SUNFLOWER OIL	30 ml
1 large	TOMATO, chopped	100 g
4 cloves	GARLIC, minced	16 g
6 pc	RED SERRANO PEPPERS, chopped	5 g
¼ cup	SALT, to prepare banana blossom	60 g
¼ cup	WHITE VINEGAR	60 ml

RECIPES AND COOKING NOTES

To taste,   SALT and PEPPER
1 large pc RED ONION, halved and
            chopped   140 g

(Serves 4)

Procedures:

1. Heat the oil in a large non-stick wok to medium heat and
    sauté garlic until golden brown in color.
2. Add the onions and cook just until they change colors.
3. Add the tomatoes and cook until soft.
4. Add the banana blossoms and peppers and stir-fry for
    a couple of minutes.
5. Pour in the vinegar and water and bring to a boil without
    mixing.
6. Reduce heat to low and simmer until water has been
    absorbed and the banana blossoms have changed
    colors and soft when pricked with a fork.
7. Season with salt and pepper and add in the vermicelli
    bean threads.
8. Gently stir in until all water has been absorbed and
    turn off the heat.

OYSTER MUSHROOM GISÁDO

Ingredients:

3 cups	OYSTER MUSHROOMS, cut into serving pieces	360 g
4 cloves	GARLIC, minced	16 g
½ pc	RED ONION, halved lengthways and sliced thinly across	60 g
2 stalks	GREEN ONIONS, chopped	20 g
1 tbsp	SUNFLOWER OIL	15 ml

85

SUSTAINING A PLANT-BASED DIET WITH FILIPINO FOOD

| 2 tbsp | VEGETARIAN STIR-FRY SAUCE | 30 ml |

(Serves 3)

Procedures:

1. In a non-stick wok, heat the oil to medium heat.
2. Sauté the garlic until golden brown in color.
3. Add the onions and cook just until they change colors.
4. Stir-in the sauce and wait until it is thoroughly heated.
5. Add the oyster mushrooms and coat thoroughly with the sauce.
6. Turn off the heat, add the green onions and continue mixing in the heat source. Rest for five minutes.

EGGPLANT INÍHAW WITH COCONUT MILK

Ingredients:

6 pc	EGGPLANTS	860 g
1 large pc	RED ONION, chopped	120 g
2 tbsp	WHITE VINEGAR	30 ml
To taste,	SALT and PEPPER	
1 cup	COCONUT CREAM	250 ml

(Serves 2)

Procedures:

1. Wash and clean the eggplants in running water and wipe with kitchen towel.
2. Pierce the eggplant skins in several places to keep them from bursting from too much contained heat.

RECIPES AND COOKING NOTES

3. Broil the eggplants over hot charcoals or in an oven toaster at 240°C, or 460°F for twenty to twenty-five minutes.
4. When cooked, peel the eggplants and chop finely.
5. Place the chopped eggplants, onions and coconut cream in a wok and bring to a boil to medium heat.
6. Season with salt and pepper and serve hot.

CHEESY PIMIENTO SPREAD

Ingredients:

1 cup	UNSALTED CASHEW NUTS	150 g
½ cup	WATER	125 ml
3 tbsp	NUTRITIONAL YEAST FLAKES	45 g
1 large pc	RED PIMIENTO PEPPER	110 g
1 tsp	SALT	5 g
2 tsp	MAPLE SYRUP	10 ml

Procedures:

1. Broil the pimiento pepper in an over toaster for twenty to twenty-five minutes and chop finely.
2. Soak the nuts in water for six hours.
3. Blend in water until smooth and transfer into a mixing bowl.
4. Add the rest of the ingredients and store in an airtight container and refrigerate until needed.

SUSTAINING A PLANT-BASED DIET WITH FILIPINO FOOD

KANGKÓNG ADÓBO

Ingredients:

3 bundles	KANGKÓNG, leaves separated from hard stems	300 g
3 tbsp	SOY SAUCE	45 ml
3 tbsp	WHITE VINEGAR	45 ml
1 tbsp	COCONUT SUGAR	15 ml
4 cloves	GARLIC, minced	16 g

(Serves 2)

Procedures:

1. Wash the kangkóng thoroughly.
2. Using a salad spinner, dry the washed kangkóng to avoid too much splatter during cooking.
3. Sauté the garlic until golden brown in color.
4. Add the stems first and stir-fry for two minutes until they turn light in color.
5. Add the vinegar and bring to a boil.
6. Season with soy sauce and coconut sugar.
7. Add the leaves during the last minute of cooking and mix well.

SNAKE BEANS ADÓBO

Ingredients:

1½ tbsp	SUNFLOWER OIL	22 ml
1 large pc	RED ONION, halved lengthways and sliced thinly across	120 g
6 cloves	GARLIC, minced	24 g
2 pc	GREEN CHILLI PEPPERS	60 g

½ cup	WHITE VINEGAR	125 ml
¼ cup	SOY SAUCE	60 ml
1 tbsp	VEGETARIAN STIR-FRY SAUCE	15 ml
¼ cup	WATER	65 ml
1 bundle	SNAKE BEANS, stringed and cut into 3-inch pieces	300 g
1 cup	TOFU, fried and cut into ½ inch cubes	250 g

(Serves 3)

Procedures:

1. Heat oil in a non-stick wok to medium and sauté the garlic until golden brown in color.
2. Add the onions and cook just until they change colors.
3. Pour in the vinegar, soy sauce, stir-fry sauce and water and bring to a boil.
4. Reduce heat to simmer and add the snake beans and green chilli peppers.
5. Cook uncovered for seven to ten minutes.
6. Add the fried tofu and continue cooking for five more minutes.
7. Taste and check the seasonings.

BAMBOO SHOOT ADÓBO

Ingredients:

1 can	BAMBOO SHOOT HALVES IN WATER, drained and sliced	540 g
1 cup	SWEET POTATOES, cut into 1½-inch cubes	180 g
6 cloves	GARLIC, minced	24 g
¼ cup	WHITE VINEGAR	60 ml

SUSTAINING A PLANT-BASED DIET WITH FILIPINO FOOD

2 tbsp	LIGHT SOY SAUCE	30 ml
1 tbsp	VEGETARIAN OYSTER MUSHROOM SAUCE	15 ml
1 tbsp	SUNFLOWER OIL	15 ml
½ pc	VEGETABLE STOCK CUBE,	5 g
1 cup	WATER	250 ml
1 pc	RED ONION, chopped	160 g

(Serves 3)

Procedures:

1. Heat the oil in a large cooking pot, heat the oil to medium heat and sauté the garlic until golden brown in color.
2. Add the onions and cook just until they change colors.
3. Pour in the water, white vinegar, soy sauce and the vegetarian oyster mushroom sauce.
4. When the liquid is starting to boil, stir in the vegetable stock cube until it is dissolved.
5. When the adobo mixture reaches a rolling boil, reduce heat to simmer and add the bamboo shoots and the sweet potatoes.
6. Cook uncovered until only a thick sauce remains of the liquid. Stir the sauce to cover the vegetable.
7. Turn off heat and rest the dish in the heat source until ready to serve.

MUNG BEANS WITH BITTER GOURD LEAVES GISÁDO

Ingredients:

1 cup, dry	COOKED MUNG BEANS	200 g
3 cups	BITTER GOURD LEAVES or ampalayá leaves, sorted	

RECIPES AND COOKING NOTES

	with hard stems removed	45 g
3 cups	PUMPKIN or *kalabása,* cut into	
	1-inch cubes	520 g
1 pc	VEGETABLE STOCK CUBE,	
	chicken-style	10 g
2 cups	WATER	500 ml
2 tbsp	SUNFLOWER OIL	30 ml
4 cloves	GARLIC, minced	16 g
1 large pc	TOMATO, chopped	70 g
To taste,	LIGHT SOY SAUCE	
To taste,	COARSELY GROUND BLACK PEPPER	
1 large pc	RED ONION, chopped	120 g

(Serves 4)

Procedures:

1. Clean and rinse the mung beans in running water for several minutes.
2. Cover them in clean tap water and soak for at least an hour before cooking.
3. Transfer the soaked mung beans in a small cooking pot and change the soaking water with clean water to cook.
4. Bring the pot to a boil to medium heat.
5. When the water reaches a rolling boil, reduce heat to low. Cooking mung beans to high heat will cause the liquid to be too starchy.
6. When the bean skins show signs of cracking, turn off the heat.
7. Heat the oil in a large cooking pot to medium heat and sauté the garlic until golden brown in color.
8. Add the onions and cook just until they change colors.
9. Add the chopped tomato and cook until soft.
10. Stir in the pumpkin cubes and cook for two minutes before adding the cooked mung beans.
11. Pour in the water and crush the vegetable stock cube in with the mixture.

SUSTAINING A PLANT-BASED DIET WITH FILIPINO FOOD

12. When the mixture reaches a rolling boil, reduce heat to simmer.
13. Continue cooking, uncovered, for ten to fifteen minutes, stirring occasionally.
14. Season with light soy sauce and coarsely ground black pepper.
15. Add the bitter gourd leaves and cook for another two minutes before turning off the heat.

BAMBOO SHOOT GISÁDO

Ingredients:

1 can	BAMBOO SHOOTS IN BRINE, drained, rinsed and pressed	560 g
1 cup	TOFU, cut into 1-inch cubes, fried	200 g
½ pc	VEGETABLE STOCK CUBE	5 g
1 small pc	RED ONION, chopped	90 g
4 cloves	GARLIC, minced	16 g
3 small pc	TOMATOES, chopped	75 g
2 tbsp	SUNFLOWER OIL	30 ml
To taste,	LIGHT SOY SAUCE, SALT and PEPPER	
¾ cup	WATER	175 ml

(Serves 2)

Procedures:

1. Heat oil in a non-stick wok to medium heat and sauté the garlic until golden brown in color.
2. Add the onions and cook just until they change colors.
3. Add the tomatoes and cook until soft.
4. Add the fried tofu and stir-fry for two minutes.
5. Pour the vegetable stock and bring to a boil.

RECIPES AND COOKING NOTES

6. Reduce heat to low and simmer for an additional two minutes.
7. Add the bamboo shoots and season with soy sauce, salt and pepper.
8. Cook until the bamboo shoots are tender.

CABBAGE AND CARROTS GISÁDO

Ingredients:

1 small pc	CABBAGE, sliced thinly	600 g
1 large pc	CARROT, peeled and julienned	150 g
4 cloves	GARLIC, minced	16 g
1 large pc	TOMATO, chopped	100 g
¼ pc	VEGETABLE STOCK CUBE, chicken-style	2.5 g
¼ cup	WATER	60 ml
1 tbsp	SUNFLOWER OIL	15 ml
2 tbsp	VEGETARIAN STIR-FRY SAUCE	30 ml
1 large pc	RED ONION, halved lengthways and sliced thinly across	140 g

(Serves 3)

Procedures:

1. Heat the oil in a non-stick wok to medium heat and sauté the garlic until golden brown in color.
2. Add the onions and cook just until they change colors.
3. Add the tomatoes and cook until soft.
4. Add water, vegetable stock cube and stir-fry sauce.
5. When the sauté mixture is boiling briskly, add the cabbage slices and carrot pieces.
6. Cover and cook until tender.

SUSTAINING A PLANT-BASED DIET WITH FILIPINO FOOD

MUSHROOM AND BOK CHOY GISÁDO

Ingredients:

2 bundles	BOK CHOY, hard stems cut-off and leaves separated and washed	300 g
1 pack	BUTTON MUSHROOMS, sliced	300 g
4 cloves	GARLIC, minced	12 g
1 small pc	RED ONION, halved lengthways and sliced thinly across	90 g
1 tsp	GINGER, cut into small sticks	5 g
2 tbsp	VEGETARIAN OYSTER MUSHROOM SAUCE	30 ml
2 tbsp	WATER	30 ml
2 tbsp	SUNFLOWER OIL	30 ml

(Serves 2)

Procedures:

1. Heat the oil in a non-stick wok to medium heat and sauté the garlic until golden brown in color.
2. Add the onions and the ginger and cook just until they change colors and fragrant.
3. Pour in the stir-fry sauce and the water and wait until it begins to boil.
4. Add the bok choy leaves and cook until it is slightly wilted in the sauce.
5. Add the mushrooms and cook for two more minutes before turning of the heat.
6. Continue with the stir-fry to mix everything well before transferring to a serving plate.

RECIPES AND COOKING NOTES

TAHÔ WITH TAPIOCA PEARLS

Ingredients:

1 block	SILKEN TOFU	450 g
½ cup, dry	SMALL TAPIOCA PEARLS	120 g
½ cup	MAPLE SYRUP	125 ml
¼ cup	SESAME SEEDS, toasted	60 g

(Serves 3)

Procedures:

1. Cook the tapioca pearls according to package instruction. Cool and set aside.
2. In a non-stick wok, toast the sesame seeds to medium heat for five minutes or just until they are lightly browned. Set aside.
3. In a small steamer, bring enough water to a boil to medium heat.
4. When the water reaches a rolling boil, reduce heat to low and add the silken tofu.
5. Steam to cook for ten minutes, turn off the heat and leave the tofu in the heat source for five more minutes.
6. Transfer to an appropriate container and add the tapioca pearls and the maple syrup.
7. Chill before serving.

EGGPLANT BISTÉK

Ingredients:

5-6 pc	EGGPLANTS, halved lengthwise	500 g

SUSTAINING A PLANT-BASED DIET WITH FILIPINO FOOD

2 tbsp	LEMON or *kalamansî* juice	30 ml
2 tbsp	SOY SAUCE	30 ml
2 tsp	MAPLE SYRUP	10 ml
2 tbsp	WATER	30 ml
2 tbsp	SUNFLOWER OIL	30 ml
To taste,	SALT and PEPPER	
	OLIVE OIL SPRAY	
1 large pc	RED ONION, cut into rings	150 g

(Serves 4)

Procedures:

1. Heat a non-stick frying pan to low to medium heat.
2. When heated, spray with olive oil spray and fry the eggplant pieces until the flesh side turns dark brown in color. Set aside.
3. Heat a non-stick wok to medium heat and add the sunflower oil.
4. Stir-fry the onion rings just until they change colors and set them aside.
5. Add the lemon juice, soy sauce, maple syrup and water and bring to a boil.
6. Season with salt and pepper.
7. When the sauce is reduced and has thickened slightly, add in the fried eggplants.
8. Bring the dish to a boil and turn off the heat. Add the onion rings and serve.

LEAFY GREENS WITH STIR-FRY SAUCE

Ingredients:

2 bundles	CHOY SUM, stems cut-off	300 g
2 bundles	BOK CHOY, stems cut-off	300 g

RECIPES AND COOKING NOTES

2 bundles	KANGKÓNG, leaves separated from hard stems	200 g
¼ cup	VEGETARIAN OYSTER MUSHROOM SAUCE	60 ml
1 tbsp	SUNFLOWER OIL, optional	15 g

(Serves 3)

Procedures:

1. Cut off the stems of choy sum and bok choy about two inches from the base of the green leaves.
2. Cut off all good leaves from hard stems of kangkóng and keep the young leaves on softer stems.
3. Clean the sorted leaves in running water and use a salad spinner to dry the leaves.
4. Put enough water to blanch the leafy vegetables in a stock pot and bring to a boil to medium heat. Add the sunflower oil if desired.
5. When the water reaches a rolling boil, reduce heat to medium and add the washed leaves and begin timing the blanch for a full minute.
6. Drain the water in a pasta strainer or sieve and transfer to a serving platter.
7. Mix in the vegetarian oyster mushroom sauce and oil, if desired. Serve hot.

LÁING

Ingredients:

5 cups	DRIED TARO LEAVES	100 g
1 pack	VEGGIE SAUSAGES, cut into 2-inch pieces	300 g
1 tbsp	VEGETARIAN OYSTER MUSHROOM	

SUSTAINING A PLANT-BASED DIET WITH FILIPINO FOOD

	SAUCE	15 ml
4 cloves	GARLIC, minced	16 g
3 cups	COCONUT MILK	750 ml
2 cups	COCONUT CREAM	500 ml
1 tbsp	GINGER, crushed	20 g
4 pc	GREEN CHILLI PEPPERS, cut	
	into ½-inch pieces	80 g
6 pc	SERRANO PEPPERS, sliced thinly	14 g
2 cups	TARO, cut into 1½-inch cubes	300 g
1 tbsp	SUNFLOWER OIL	15 g
1 pc	RED ONION, quartered	120 g

(Serves 4)

Procedures:

1. Heat the oil in a cooking pot to medium heat and sauté the garlic until golden brown in color.
2. Add the onions and ginger and cook until the onions are soft and the aroma starts to fill the air.
3. Add the veggie sausages and the taro and stir-fry for two minutes.
4. Pour in the coconut milk and the oyster mushroom sauce and bring to a boil.
5. Add the dried taro leaves and with the back of a ladle weight it down to absorb the coconut milk. It is important to remember **not** to stir the pot.
6. Reduce the heat to simmer and let the leaves cook until all coconut milk has been absorbed.
7. Add and press down the chillies and pour in the coconut cream.
8. Cook until all the coconut cream has been absorbed by the taro leaves and the leaves are soft enough to chew.
9. Turn off heat.
10. Cover and leave in the heat source for several minutes to further reduce the sauce before serving.

ENSALÁDANG PILIPÍNO

Traditional Filipino salads are not really salads but a combination of pre-cooked vegetables that are blended together by one common flavor which is more of a dipping sauce than a salad dressing.

Ingredients:

4–5 pc	LONG EGGPLANTS, pierced	600 g
1 pc	GREEN BELL PEPPER	190 g
1 pc	RED BELL PEPPER	190 g
10 pc	ÓKRA LADY FINGER	100 g
1 small pc	BITTER GOURD	140 g
5 pc	SNAKE BEANS, cut into 2-inch long pieces	120 g
1 bundle	SWEET POTATO TOPS, sorted with hard stems taken off	140 g
3 pc	TOMATOES, sliced	300 g
To taste,	LIGHT SOY SAUCE	
1 large pc	RED ONION, halved lengthways and sliced thinly across	180 g

(Serves 3)

Procedures:

1. Wash all the vegetables thoroughly and separate the eggplants and peppers from the rest. Remember to pierce the eggplants with a fork in different parts to prevent them from bursting from too much contained heat.
2. Set the oven toaster to highest setting at twenty minutes and arrange the eggplants and bell peppers, making sure there is ample space between each one.
3. Put enough water in a stock pot, add a teaspoon of salt and heat to medium.

SUSTAINING A PLANT-BASED DIET WITH FILIPINO FOOD

4. When the water reaches a rolling boil, carefully put in the vegetables one kind at a time.
5. Different vegetables require varied cooking times, so keep watch so as not to overcook of any of them.
6. Generally, sweet potato tops cook first, bitter gourd will be second, and okra, third. Snake beans will take longest to cook.
7. When cooked, cut the vegetables in serving pieces and arrange in a platter.
8. Season the tomatoes and toss in the sliced raw onions and serve as a dip.
9. You can also serve them with vinegar dip, if desired.

PICO DE GALLO

Ingredients:

2 pc	RED ONIONS, diced	380 g
5–6 pc	TOMATOES, barely ripe	500 g
1 cup	FRESH CILANTRO LEAVES	90 g
3 pc	JALAPEÑO PEPPERS	120 g
1 pc	LIME	40 g
To taste,	TABLE SALT	

(Serves 4)

Ingredients:

1. In a mixing bowl, dice the onions and tomatoes finely and add the cilantro leaves to the mix.
2. Cut the jalapeño peppers in half, deseed and chop finely. Add to the diced onions and tomatoes.
3. Slice the lime and squeeze its juice on the diced vegetables.
4. Season with fine table salt.

RECIPES AND COOKING NOTES

5.   Transfer to a serving bowl and serve.

MUNG BEAN SPROUTS ENSALÁDA

Ingredients:

1 pack	FRESH MUNG BEAN SPROUTS	250 g
1 cup	BABY SPINACH LEAVES	30 g
1 pc	LEBANESE CUCUMBERS, pared and sliced	150 g
1 pc	CARROT, julienned	150 g
2 tbsp	PINE NUTS	30 g
2 tbsp	WHITE VINEGAR	30 ml
2 tbsp	WATER	30 ml
2 tbsp	COCONUT SUGAR	30 ml
To taste,	COARSELY GROUND BLACK PEPPER	

(Serves 3)

Procedures:

1.   For the dressing, combine the vinegar, water sugar and ground black pepper together. Make sure the sugar is well dissolved. Set aside.
2.   Sort the fresh mung bean sprouts for spoils and cut the root tips.
3.   Wash the baby spinach leaves in running water and dry in a salad spinner.
4.   Combine all the salad ingredients in a serving bowl and drizzle with the vinegar dressing.

CARROTS AND ROUND BEANS ENSALÁDA

Ingredients:

1 pc	CARROT	120 g
12 pc	ROUND BEANS	100 g
Dash of	COARSELY GROUND BLACK PEPPER	
3 tbsp	PINE NUTS	45 g
3 tbsp	DRIED CRANBERRIES	40 g
¼ cup	BALSAMIC VINEGAR	60 ml
3 tbsp	LIGHT SOY SAUCE	45 ml
2 tsp	MAPLE SYRUP	10 ml
1 pc	RED ONION, halved and sliced thinly	100 g

(Serves 2)

Procedures:

1. Using a papaya grater, grate the carrot into long thin strands. Alternatively, you can also cut it into small matchstick-size pieces.
2. Heat two cups of water in a small cooking pot to high heat.
3. Blanch the beans for one minute and rinse in a wire sieve over running water to cool and stop it from cooking.
4. Slice the beans into thin diagonal slices.
5. Mix the carrots, beans, cranberries and pine nuts and onions together.
6. Mix the balsamic vinegar, light soy sauce and maple syrup and drizzle over the prepared salad vegetables.

RECIPES AND COOKING NOTES

CAULIFLOWER ENSALÁDA

Ingredients:

1 small pc	CAULIFLOWER, cut into florets	360 g
1 big pc	RED ONION, halved and finely chopped	160 g
1 small pc	GREEN BELL PEPPER, deseeded and cut into strips	220 g
2 pc	ROMA TOMATOES, cut into wedges	130 g
1 tsp	SEA SALT	5 g
4 cups	WATER	1 L
2 tbsp	PEPITAS	30 g

(Serves 4)

Procedures:

1. Heat the water together with the salt in a cooking pot to medium heat.
2. When the water reaches a rolling boil, reduce heat to medium and add the cauliflower florets and start watching from two minutes of blanching. The florets must retain a crisp when done.
3. Drain the pot in a wire sieve under running water to stop the florets from cooking. Cool and drain thoroughly then transfer to a serving bowl.
4. Add the onions, bell pepper strips, tomatoes and pepitas and drizzle with mustard and maple syrup dressing.

Mustard & Maple Syrup Dressing

Ingredients:

¼ cup	DIJON MUSTARD	60 g
3 tbsp	MAPLE SYRUP	45 g

SUSTAINING A PLANT-BASED DIET WITH FILIPINO FOOD

Procedure:

- Mix the ingredients together and use as dressing.

BITTER GOURD TOMATO ENSALÁDA

Ingredients:

1 large pc	BITTER GOURD	350 g
To taste,	SEA SALT	
1 large pc	RED ONION, sliced thinly	120 g
12 pc	CHERRY TOMATOES, halved	80 g

(Serves 3)

Procedures:

1. Cut the bitter gourd in half along the grain and scrape off the seeds.
2. Slice the halves across into thin slices.
3. Rub the sliced bitter gourd with salt and let it stand for ten minutes.
4. Squeeze manually to remove both the salt and the bitter taste.
5. Rinse with water and squeeze out the liquid.
6. In a serving bowl, combine the bitter gourd with the onions and tomatoes.
7. Drizzle with the oil-free Balsamic Vinegar salad dressing.
8. Chill and serve.

Balsamic Vinegar Dressing

Ingredients:

RECIPES AND COOKING NOTES

¼ cup	BALSAMIC VINEGAR	60 ml
3 tbsp	LIGHT SOY SAUCE	45 ml
1 tbsp	MAPLE SYRUP	15 ml
Dash of	COARSELY GROUND BLACK PEPPER	

Procedure:

- Mix all ingredients together making sure the syrup is well dissolved.

BOILING SWEET POTATOES

The traditional way we were taught of boiling sweet potatoes can be helpful when cooking this nutritious root crop away from home. This is particularly true when the available varieties happen to contain too much water such as the gold and white sweet potato types.

Cook these types in a heavy-set pot with very little water—start with as low as a fourth of an inch to cover the bottom of the pot—arrange the roots well and cover with a clean tea-towel or cheesecloth before closing with the pot cover.

Check from twenty minutes of cooking but they will usually be done in thirty minutes.

SUSTAINING A PLANT-BASED DIET WITH FILIPINO FOOD

USING FROZEN CORN KERNELS

Frozen corn kernels are raw corn that are mechanically removed from the cob immediately after harvest and snap or blast-frozen with cool air to preserve their freshness.

Using frozen corn kernels that are uncooked, directly from the freezer or even thawed afterwards adds unwanted water from the liquid that's been collected within the cereals during the freezing process.

Frozen corn kernels need to be pre-cooked before they can be added to any recipe. However, they usually require less time to cook than fresh corn on the cob.

The approximate cooking time for boiling frozen corn kernels is ten to fifteen minutes. Adding a bit of salt while boiling will do much to improve the flavor of the cereal.

Steaming to cook frozen corn kernels will take from fifteen to twenty minutes before they are ready.

OVEN-ROASTED VEGETABLES WITH GARDEN ENSALÁDA

Ingredients:

1 cup	SWEET POTATOES, cut into ¾-inch cubes	150 g
1 cup	BUTTERNUT PUMPKIN, cut into ¾-inch cubes	140 g
1 cup	CARROTS, cut into ¾-inch cubes	90 g

RECIPES AND COOKING NOTES

1 cup	CORN KERNELS, cooked	150 g
1 pack	SPICE MIX (Mexican Chipotle, Caldereta Mix or Moroccan Spices)	57 g
1 cup	BABY SPINACH LEAVES	30 g
1 pc	LEBANESE CUCUMBERS, pared and sliced	150 g
1 pc	CARROT, julienned	150 g
2 tbsp	PINE NUTS	30 g
1 large pc	RED ONION, halved across and sliced thinly	180 g
¼ cup	DIJON MUSTARD	60 g
3 tbsp	MAPLE SYRUP	45 ml

(Serves 4)

Procedures:

1. Combine the dijon mustard and maple syrup well and set aside.
2. Preheat oven to 180°C, or 350°F.
3. In a mixing bowl, spread the seasonings evenly among the sweet potatoes, butternut pumpkin and carrot cubes.
4. Line a baking tray with baking paper and arrange the diced vegetables.
5. Set the time to thirty minutes but start watching out from twenty minutes of baking as cooking times vary for different ovens.
6. When done, take out of the oven and cool for five minutes in the baking tray before transferring to a serving plate.
7. Add the baby spinach leaves, lebanese cucumbers, carrots, corn kernels and pine nuts.
8. Toss In the raw sliced onions.
9. Drizzle with dijon mustard and maple syrup dressing.

SUSTAINING A PLANT-BASED DIET WITH FILIPINO FOOD

BARBECUE BROAD BEANS AND CHICKPEAS

Ingredients:

½ cup	DRIED BROAD BEANS, partially cooked	100 g
½ cup	DRIED LIMA BEANS, partially cooked	110 g
½ cup	DRIED CHICKPEAS, partially cooked	90 g
½ cup	SOY SAUCE	125 ml
6 tbsp	LEMON JUICE or *kalamansî* juice	90 ml
¼ cup	COCONUT SUGAR	60 g
8 cloves	GARLIC, crushed	32 g
2 pc	SERRANO PEPPERS, chopped	2 g
1 tbsp	SUNFLOWER OIL	15 ml
½ cup	WATER	125 ml

(Serves 4)

Procedures:

1. Soak the beans and the chickpeas overnight and discard the soaking water.
2. Sort and discard discolored and deformed lima beans and chickpeas.
3. Peel the broad beans by squeezing each one   between thumb and forefinger.
4. Heat enough water, keeping in mind they will expand to approximately three times their sizes after they are soaked, in an appropriately-sized cooking pot to medium heat.
5. When the water reaches a rolling boil, reduce heat to simmer and cook the beans and chickpeas for thirty minutes. Drain well.

RECIPES AND COOKING NOTES

6. In another cooking pot, combine the soy sauce, lemon juice, coconut sugar, garlic, peppers, sunflower oil and water.
7. Set heat to low to medium heat and let it cook for fifteen minutes uncovered.
8. Add the partially cooked beans in the cooked barbecue seasonings and cook for an additional twenty minutes, stirring occasionally for the beans to be evenly seasoned.
9. Continue cooking this way until all the liquid has been absorbed by the beans and until they retain a shiny appearance.

LIMA BEANS SINIGÁNG

Ingredients:

2 pc	RED ONIONS, quartered	240 g
2 pc	RIPE TOMATOES, sliced	200 g
½ tbsp	GINGER, slivered	8 g
½ pack	TAMARIND SOUP BASE MIX	20 g
4 cups	WATER	1 L
2 packs	VEGETABLE STOCK CUBES	20 g
1 cup, dry	LIMA BEANS, partially cooked for 50 minutes	200 g
4 pc	GREEN CHILLI PEPPERS	80 g
12 pc	OKRA, stem cut-off	160 g
12 pc	SNAKE BEANS or *sitáw*, cut into 3-inch long pieces	240 g
2–3 pc	TARO or *gábe*, peeled and cut into 2-inch cubes	400 g
1 bundle	KANGKÓNG, tough stems cut-off	300 g
2 pc	BOK CHOY or *pétsay*, leaves separated	320 g
To taste,	SALT and PEPPER	

SUSTAINING A PLANT-BASED DIET WITH FILIPINO FOOD

(Serves 5)

Procedures:

1. Soak the lima beans in filtered water overnight.
2. Discard the soaking water and rinse the lima beans in running water.
3. Pour a liter and a half of filtered water in a cooking pot and add the lima beans.
4. Bring to a boil to high heat. Reduce to medium heat when the liquid reaches a rolling boil.
5. Cook the lima beans for fifty minutes.
6. Drain in a wire sieve and discard the unusable beans.
7. In a large cooking pot, combine water, red onions, tomatoes, ginger, tamarind soup base mix and vegetable stock cubes.
8. Bring to a boil to medium heat and continue cooking until tomatoes have wilted and the soup has slightly changed colors.
9. Add the partially cooked lima beans, taro and green chilli peppers.
10. When the soup has resumed boiling, continue cooking for ten to fifteen more minutes before adding the snake beans.
11. Wait for the soup to boil again and cook for five more minutes before adding the okra and the kangkóng with bigger stems and boil for two more minutes.
12. Season with salt and pepper and add the kangkóng leaves and bok choy.
13. Turn off the heat and leave covered until served.

RECIPES AND COOKING NOTES

LIMA BEANS WITH SWEET POTATOES GISÁDO

Ingredients:

2 cups	LIMA BEANS, cooked	190 g
6 cloves	GARLIC, minced	24 g
2 small pc	TOMATOES, sliced	200 g
2 cups	SWEET POTATOES, cut into 1-inch cubes and fried	360 g
½ pc	GREEN BELL PEPPER, diced	70 g
¼ cup	ANNATTO WATER	60 ml
½ cup	WATER	120 ml
½ pc	VEGETABLE STOCK CUBE, chicken-style	5 g
4 tbsp	SUNFLOWER OIL, halved	60 ml
2 tbsp	VEGETARIAN STIR-FRY SAUCE	30 ml
1 large pc	RED ONION, halved lengthways and sliced thinly across	150 g

(Serves 3)

Procedures:

1. Dissolve the vegetable stock cube in half a cup of water and set aside.
2. Soak a teaspoon of annatto seeds in a fourth of a cup of water for thirty minutes. Remove the seeds and set aside.
3. Heat frying pan to medium heat and add two tablespoons of the oil.
4. Fry the sweet potatoes and set aside.
5. In a non-stick wok heated to low to medium heat, add two tablespoons of the oil and sauté the garlic until golden brown in color.

111

SUSTAINING A PLANT-BASED DIET WITH FILIPINO FOOD

6. Add the onions and tomatoes and cook for one to two minutes.
7. Add the vegetable broth and bring to a boil.
8. Add the cooked lima beans, fried sweet potatoes and the bell peppers.
9. Stir in the annatto water and boil for five minutes until the sauce dish thickens.
10. Season with the vegetarian stir-fry sauce.

USING CANNED BEANS

These convenient option for a quick and nutritious meal are sadly often overlooked or are just not very popular even among purely plant-based eaters.

Straight out of the can, the contents are simply uninviting, no thanks to their apparent sloppy and sticky overall look, not to mention their plain and flavorless taste.

To improve them a bit, canned beans can be drained of the water they have been soaked in, dropped in newly-boiled liquid that has been infused with flavorings just long enough for the beans to absorb some of the liquid, drained and dried at room temperature.

Canned beans can be a stand-alone treat, served as added protein in a salad mix or added as an ingredient to a multi-ingredient viand.

RECIPES AND COOKING NOTES

CANNED BEANS SNACKS

Ingredients:

1 can	RED KIDNEY BEANS, BROWN LENTILS, BLACK BEANS or CHICKPEAS	400 g
2 cloves	GARLIC, crushed	8 g
1 pc	BAY LEAF	
Dash of	SALT	
1 pc	VEGETABLE STOCK CUBE	20 g
2 cups	WATER	500 ml

(Serves 2)

Procedures:

1. Empty the can of beans in a sieve, rinse in running water and drain thoroughly.
2. Combine all ingredients in a small saucepan and heat to boil to medium for five to seven minutes until the vegetable stock cube and the salt are completely dissolved.
3. Spoon out and discard the garlic cloves and the bay leaf.
4. Add the drained beans until the liquid reaches a rolling boil again. Turn off the heat after two minutes.
5. Rest the beans in the broth for five to ten minutes and drain to dry.
6. Serve immediately or cool and keep in the refrigerator as a quick snack option.

TOMATO BASIL PESTO

Ingredients:

2 tbsp	OLIVE OIL	30 ml
4 cloves	GARLIC, minced	16 g
2 tbsp	RED WINE VINEGAR	30 ml
3 tbsp	TOMATO PASTE	45 g
2 cans	DICED ITALIAN TOMATOES	800 g
12 pc	FRESH BASIL LEAVES or	8 g
1 tbsp	DRIED BASIL LEAVES	12 g
3 tbsp	COCONUT SUGAR	45 g
Dash of	SALT	
Dash of	COARSELY GROUND BLACK PEPPER	
3 tbsp	NUTRITIONAL YEAST FLAKES	20 g
2 tsp	GARLIC POWDER	6 g

(Serves 5)

Procedures:

1. Heat the oil in a medium saucepan to medium-low heat.
2. Add the garlic and sauté until lightly golden brown in color.
3. Add the red wine vinegar and stir for an additional two minutes.
4. Stir in the tomatoes, tomato paste, basil, maple syrup, salt and pepper.
5. Bring the mixture to a boil, reduce heat and simmer, stirring occasionally until the tomatoes break down.
6. Remove the saucepan from heat and cool slightly.
7. Place the sauce, nutritional yeast flakes and garlic powder in a small food processor and pulse until smooth.

RECIPES AND COOKING NOTES

WHITE BEANS WITH TOMATO PESTO

Ingredients:

2 cups	DRIED CANNELLINI BEANS	400 g
12 cups	WATER	3 L
1 pc	BAY LEAF	
3 cloves	GARLIC	12 g
1 tsp	SALT	5 g

(Serves 3)

Procedures:

1. Clean the dried beans in running water several times until water appears clear when the beans are left to soak for some time.
2. Make sure the beans are well submerged in water and soak the beans for at least six hours before cooking.
3. In a large cooking pot, bring the water to a boil to high heat.
4. When the water reaches a rolling boil, reduce heat to medium and drop in the beans, bay leaf and garlic.
5. Cook uncovered, stir occasionally and monitor the water level.
6. Start checking from fifty minutes of cooking. Add the salt.
7. When the beans reach the desired softness, turn off heat.
8. Drain well in pasta strainer and transfer to a serving platter.
9. Serve with tomato basil pesto from the preceding recipe.

SUSTAINING A PLANT-BASED DIET WITH FILIPINO FOOD

PASTA WITH TOMATO PESTO

Ingredients:

2 cups	FUSILLI PASTA	210 ml
6 cups	WATER	1.5 L
1 tbsp	SALT	15 g
1 tbsp	SUNFLOWER OIL	15 ml

(Serves 3)

Procedures:

1. In a stockpot, bring water to a boil to high heat.
2. When the water reaches a rolling boil, add the salt and oil and reduce heat to medium.
3. Cook as directed in the package instruction.
4. Drain in a pasta sieve or colander and cool down with running water to stop it from cooking. Pasta should be *al dente* when done.
5. Drain well before serving.
6. Serve with tomato basil pesto from the preceding recipe.

PESTO PIZZA

The Tomato Basil Pesto recipe from the previous page can be used as a pizza sauce for this pizza. You may also use the accompanying pizza sauce recipe described below.

Pizza Base

Ingredients:

½ cup	WHOLEMEAL FLOUR	80 g
½ cup	OAT FLOUR	60 g

116

RECIPES AND COOKING NOTES

½ tsp	DRIED BASIL LEAVES	3 g
½ cup	WATER	120 ml
¼ tsp	SALT	2 g

(Serves 3)

Procedures:

1. With the use of a rubber scraper, mix all ingredients together in a small mixing bowl. The mixture will be runny.
2. Preheat a twelve-inch non-stick frying pan to high heat.
3. Grease with olive oil spray when it is sufficiently hot.
4. Scrape out the mixture into the center of the hot frying pan and tilt the pan to make a nine-inch flat bread.
5. Reduce heat to medium and wait until the sides of the flat bread are well dried out and firm.
6. Alternatively, you may use a rubber scraper to lift from the sides to see if the bottom part touching the frying pan is cooked to your liking.
7. Turn the flat bread over with one flip, as if turning over a pancake.
8. When done, turn off heat and transfer the pizza base to a cake cooler.

Pizza Sauce

Ingredients:

1 cup	TOMATO SAUCE	250 ml
1 tub	TOMATO PASTE	140 g
3 tbsp	COCONUT SUGAR	45 g
3 cloves	GARLIC, minced	12 g
1 large pc	RED ONION, chopped	130 g
To taste,	SALT and PEPPER	
1 tbsp	DRIED BASIL LEAVES	15 g
½ tbsp	DRIED OREGANO LEAVES	8 g
1 tsp	DRIED THYME LEAVES	5 g

SUSTAINING A PLANT-BASED DIET WITH FILIPINO FOOD

1 tbsp	OLIVE OIL	15 ml

Procedures:

1. In a cooking pot, heat the olive oil to high heat.
2. Reduce heat to low-medium heat and sauté the garlic until golden brown in color.
3. Add the chopped onion and cook just until the pieces have changed colors.
4. Pour in the tomato sauce.
5. When the tomato sauce begins to boil add the basil, oregano and thyme leaves. Reduce heat to low, cover and cook for ten minutes.
6. Add the tomato paste and the coconut sugar and stir well to mix the sauce thoroughly.
7. Cook uncovered for five more minutes and turn off the heat.

Toppings

Ingredients:

1 pc	GREEN BELL PEPPER, sliced into rings	180 g
1 pc	RED ONION, sliced into rings	120 g
½ cup	BASIL LEAVES	25 g
½ cup	BUTTON MUSHROOMS, sliced	80 g
1 tbsp	NUTRITIONAL YEAST FLAKES	15 g

Procedures:

1. Lightly brush the pizza base with olive oil.
2. Spread the nutritional yeast flakes evenly.
3. With a rubber scraper, spread the pizza sauce of your choice on top of the nutritional yeast flakes.
4. Arrange the basil leaves on top of the pizza sauce followed by the onions, bell pepper and the button mushrooms.

RECIPES AND COOKING NOTES

5. Preheat oven to 180°C or 350°F.
6. Cook the pizza for fifteen to twenty minutes.

ROASTED LIMA BEANS SNACKS

Ingredients:

1 cup, dry	LIMA BEANS	200 g
1 tsp	ONION FLAKES	2 g
1 tsp	GARLIC GRANULES	2 g
1 tsp	COCONUT SUGAR	5 g
1 tsp	SESAME SEEDS	5 g
½ tsp	TABLE SALT	2 g

(Serves 3)

Procedures:

1. Soak the lima beans in filtered water overnight.
2. Discard the soaking water and rinse the beans in running water.
3. Pour a liter and a half of filtered water in a cooking pot and add the lima beans.
4. Bring to a boil to high heat.
5. When the water reaches a rolling boil, reduce heat to medium and cook the lima beans for an hour and a half.
6. Drain in a wire sieve.
7. Pat dry with kitchen towels and air dry while preheating the oven.
8. Preheat oven to 220°C or 425°F.
9. Arrange the lima beans on a baking tray and bake for fifty minutes, stirring occasionally.
10. Let the lima beans rest in the tray for ten minutes.
11. Remove to a bowl.

SUSTAINING A PLANT-BASED DIET WITH FILIPINO FOOD

12. Using a marble mortar and pestle, pulverize the onion flakes, garlic granules, sesame seeds and table salt together.
13. Add the coconut sugar and mix well.
14. Sprinkle on lima beans and serve.

AMPALAYÁ SMOOTHIE

Ingredients:

1 pc	BANANA, cut into small pieces	170 g
1 pc	CARROT, sliced thinly	110 g
1 small pc	RED DELICIOUS APPLE , quartered, cored and sliced thinly	190 g
1 small pc	BITTER GOURD, halved and sliced thinly	180 g
2 stalks	CELERY, sliced thinly	140 g
1 pc	LEBANESE CUCUMBER, sliced	120 g
3 cups	KALE, hard stems discarded, leaves finely shredded	300 g
1 tbsp	FLAXSEED MEAL	15 g
1½ cups	PINEAPPLE JUICE	375 ml
1½ cups	LIGHT SOY MILK	375 ml

(Serves 4)

Procedures:

1. In a 1.5 liter blender, pulse together all ingredients until smooth.
2. Pour into a pitcher and keep in the refrigerator, where it will keep fresh for three days, until needed.

RECIPES AND COOKING NOTES

CREAMED CORN AND SPLIT PEA SUWÁM

Ingredients:

1 can	CREAMED CORN	420 g
½ cup, dry	GREEN SPLIT PEAS, partially cooked for forty-five minutes	125 g
2 tbsp	SUNFLOWER OIL	30 ml
4 cloves	GARLIC, minced	16 g
1 tsp	SEA SALT	5 g
Dash of	BLACK PEPPER	
½ pc	VEGETABLE STOCK CUBE, chicken-style	5 g
1 cup	WATER	250 ml
1 cup	MORINGA or *malúnggay* leaves	45 g
½ cup	PEPPER LEAVES	10 g
½ cup	FRIED GARLIC, to serve	48 g
1 pc	RED ONION, halved lengthwise and sliced thinly	120 g

(Serves 4)

Procedures:

1. In a wire sieve, clean and rinse the split peas in running water.
2. Transfer to a small cooking pot and add enough water to cover with an extra two inches above the peas.
3. Heat the pot to medium heat and bring to a boil.
4. When the pot reaches a rolling boil, reduce heat to simmer for 45–50 minutes, adding water as necessary.
5. When the peas are partially cooked, turn off the heat and set them aside.
6. Heat the oil in a cooking pot to medium heat.
7. Add the garlic and sauté until lightly golden brown in color.

SUSTAINING A PLANT-BASED DIET WITH FILIPINO FOOD

8. Stir in the onions and continue cooking just until they change colors.
9. Pour in the water with the vegetable stock cube, add the sea salt and black pepper and bring to a boil.
10. Continue cooking until the cube is dissolved and has combined well with the flavorings.
11. Add the creamed corn, bring to a boil and add the pre-cooked split peas.
12. Continue cooking for seven to ten more minutes or until the soup has been reduced enough and thickened.
13. Add the moringa and pepper leaves and turn off the heat.
14. Serve with the fried garlic as topping.

LENTIL AND SWEET POTATO BÓLA-BÓLA

Ingredients:

1 cup, dry	BROWN LENTILS	190 g
2 cups	COOKED SWEET POTATOES, mashed	400 g
1 pc	RED ONION, finely chopped	160 g
1 small pc	CARROT, finely chopped	90 g
3 stalks	GREEN ONIONS, finely chopped	20 g
1 tbsp	NUTRITIONAL YEAST FLAKES	7 g
To taste,	SALT and PEPPER	
3 tbsp	TAPIOCA STARCH	30 g
3 tbsp	WATER	45 ml
1 cup	WHOLEMEAL FLOUR	200 g
1 cup	SUNFLOWER OIL, to fry	250 ml

(Serves 4)

Procedures:

122

RECIPES AND COOKING NOTES

1. Dissolve the tapioca starch in water and mix until smooth. Set aside.
2. Heat a liter of water with two teaspoons salt in a cooking pot to medium heat.
3. When the water reaches a rolling boil, reduce heat to medium and add in the lentils and cook for forty-five minutes or until soft. Cool.
4. Combine lentils with mashed sweet potatoes, onions, carrots, green onions, nutritional yeast flakes and season with salt and pepper.
5. Form into balls and dip into the tapioca starch and roll in flour.
6. Arrange the prepared bola-bola in a plate or tray that has been lined with non-stick baking paper.
7. Refrigerate for at least half an hour before frying.
8. When ready, fry to golden brown as you would with meat balls.
9. Serve with ketchup or sweet chilli sauce or serve as is as they are tasty on their own.

BRAISED CARROTS AND CHAYOTE

Ingredients:

2 pc	CHAYOTE, peeled and sliced into bite-sized pieces	400 g
1 pc	CARROT, peeled and sliced diagonally	150 g
¼ pc	VEGETABLE STOCK CUBE	
½ cup	WATER	125 ml
2 pc	SHALLOTS or *sibúyas tagálog*, sliced	20 g
2 cloves	GARLIC, crushed	8 g
Dash of	SALT and PEPPER	

SUSTAINING A PLANT-BASED DIET WITH FILIPINO FOOD

(Serves 3)

Procedures:

1. In a cooking pot, dissolve the vegetable stock cube in water and add the shallots and garlic. Season with a little salt and pepper.
2. Bring to a boil to medium heat and add the chayote and carrots.
3. Cover and cook until vegetables are tender.

SPAGHETTI WITH SWEET TOMATO SAUCE

Ingredients:

2 cans	DICED ITALIAN TOMATOES	800 g
6 cloves	GARLIC, minced	24 g
1 large pc	GREEN BELL PEPPER, diced	300 g
1 large pc	RED ONION, halved lengthways and sliced thinly across	180 g
1 cup, dry	TEXTURED VEGETABLE PROTEIN	85 g
¾ cup	HOT WATER	180 ml
½ pc	VEGETABLE STOCK CUBE, beef style	5 g
1 pack	VEGGIE SAUSAGES or VEGGIE HOTDOGS, sliced	300 g
1 tub	TOMATO PASTE	140 g
2 tbsp	DRIED BASIL LEAVES	6 g
1 tbsp	DRIED OREGANO LEAVES	3 g
2 tsp	DRIED THYME LEAVES	2 g
3 tbsp	COCONUT SUGAR	45 g
2 tbsp	SUNFLOWER OIL, to sauté	30 ml
1 tbsp	SUNFLOWER OIL, to boil pasta	15 ml
2 tsp	SEA SALT, to boil pasta	10 g
2 tbsp	NUTRITIONAL YEAST FLAKES	14 g

RECIPES AND COOKING NOTES

1 pack   WHOLEMEAL SPAGHETTI PASTA,
cooked *al dente*   750 g

(Serves 6)

Procedures:

1. In a small cooking pot dissolve the vegetable stock cube in hot water.
2. Bring to a boil quickly and turn off the heat.
3. Add the textured vegetable protein and make sure every-thing is covered by the hot liquid. Set aside and cool.
4. Put six liters of water in a large stock pot. Add sea salt and oil and bring to a boil to high heat.
5. When the water reaches a rolling boil, reduce heat to medium and add the spaghetti pasta.
6. Cook according to package instructions.
7. When cooked, drain pasta of hot water in a pasta sieve under running cold tap water to stop the pasta from cooking.
8. Drain and set aside.
9. Heat the oil in a large cooking pot to medium heat.
10. Sauté the garlic until golden brown in color.
11. Add the onions and bell peppers and cook until soft.
12. Add the cooled textured vegetable protein and the sliced vegetable sausages and the dried basil, oregano and thyme leaves.
13. Stir-fry for five to seven minutes until the meat substitutes have changed colors and the air is filled with the aroma of herbs.
14. Pour in the tomatoes, wait until the pot mixture is boiling briskly before lowering heat to simmer.
15. Cook uncovered to let the liquid escape and the sauce to thicken for ten to fifteen minutes.
16. Reduce heat to very low and add tomato paste and sugar. Mix well.
17. Cook for a further five minutes.

SUSTAINING A PLANT-BASED DIET WITH FILIPINO FOOD

18. Turn off heat and cool the sauce for at least ten minutes before adding the nutritional yeast flakes.

CHEESY OATS PÚTO

Ingredients:

1 cup	OAT FLOUR	200 g
1 cup	WHOLEMEAL FLOUR	200 g
2 tbsp	FLAXSEED MEAL	30 g
5 tbsp	HOT WATER	75 ml
1 tbsp	NUTRITIONAL YEAST FLAKES	7 g
¼ cup	MAPLE SYRUP	60 ml
2½ tsp	BAKING POWDER	12 g
½ tsp	SALT	2.5 g
1 cup	SOY MILK	250 ml

(Serves 4)

Procedures:

1. Put the flaxseed meal in a cup and add the hot but not boiling water. Mix well and let it cool down for ten minutes.
2. Put one cup of rolled oats in a blender and pulse until it turns into powder.
3. Put the oat flour in a mixing bowl together with the whole-meal flour, nutritional yeast flakes, baking powder and salt and mix well.
4. In a liquid measuring cup, mix the flaxseed liquid with the maple syrup and soy milk and pour into the flour mixture.
5. Mix well only until no more lumps can be seen when you scoop at the batter.

126

RECIPES AND COOKING NOTES

6. Grease or line the bottom of an eight-inch pie pan and pour the batter in.
7. Put enough water in a large steamer and bring to a boil to high heat.
8. When the water reaches a rolling boil, reduce heat to medium and steam the batter.
9. Start watching the cooking batter from twenty-five minutes onward. You can insert a skewer at the center to see if no more batter sticks to it. If the skewer comes out clean, the púto is cooked.
10. Turn off the heat and take the púto out and let it rest for five minutes more before serving.

SALABÁT

Ingredients:

4 tbsp	GINGER, peeled and sliced	120 g
2 pc	LEMON, halved	250 g
4 tsp	MAPLE SYRUP	20 ml
5 cups	FILTERED WATER	1.25 L

(Serves 4)

Procedures:

1. Place the peeled and sliced ginger together with the clean drinking water in a pot.
2. Bring to a boil to high heat.
3. As soon as it starts boiling, remove cover and reduce heat to very low.
4. Let it simmer for twenty minutes, turn off heat and transfer the liquid into four cups.
5. Cool for five minutes and squeeze in half a lemon in each cup of ginger tea.

SUSTAINING A PLANT-BASED DIET WITH FILIPINO FOOD

6. Sweeten each cup with a teaspoon of maple syrup and serve hot.
7. Leave the boiled ginger in the pot and pour in a cup of hot water in it. Leave to cool.
8. Discard the boiled sliced ginger before heating the salabát in the pot. Leaving it in and heating it again with the liquid will cause the drink to taste bitter.

TÁPA BITS PINÁIS WITH TURMERIC RICE

Ingredients:

1 recipe	TÁPA BITS TOPPINGS, recipe on p. 60	
4 cups	TURMERIC RICE, cooked	640 g
4 large pc	RIPE TOMATOES, cut into wedges	360 g
Dash of	SALT	
	BANANA LEAVES, to wrap	
	TIE STRINGS	

(Serves 4)

Procedures:

1. Divide the tápa from the preceding recipe into four parts and set aside.
2. Wipe the banana leaves with a clean cloth and pass through an open fire to wilt and make the leaves pliant and soft prior to wrapping.
3. Lay a prepared banana leaf on a large plate and arrange a cup of rice, the tápa and the lightly salted tomato wedges. You can manually shape the rice to better manage the sealing of your parcel.

RECIPES AND COOKING NOTES

4. Repeat with another layer of banana leaf cover to secure the dish for steaming. Tie it up with a food-grade string. Do not use plastic or synthetic strings.
5. Preheat oven to 180°C or 360°F and arrange the banana parcels on a baking tray.
6. Bake for 15 minutes and turn off the heat but leave the parcels in the oven for another five minutes.
7. Take out of the oven and serve hot.

MUNG BEANS WITH MAPLE SOY MILK

Ingredients:

1 cup, dry	MUNG BEANS	210 g
2 cups	SOY MILK	500 ml
6 tsp	MAPLE SYRUP	30 ml

(Serves 3)

Procedures:

1. Place the mung beans in a wire sieve and pass through running water.
2. Soak the mung beans for at least an hour before cooking. Discard the water that has been used to soak the beans.
3. Put fresh water in a cooking pot and stir in the mung beans.
4. Heat the pot to medium heat.
5. When the water begins to boil, reduce heat to very low to cook the mung beans.
6. Cooking mung beans to high heat will cause the liquid to be starchy.

SUSTAINING A PLANT-BASED DIET WITH FILIPINO FOOD

7. When the skins of the beans begin to crack, turn off the heat but leave the cooking pot in the heat source for the beans to continue cooking.
8. Serve the cooked mung beans with soy milk and maple syrup as a snacking option.

BANANA OATS MARUYÀ

Ingredients:

2 large pc	RIPE BANANAS, mashed	300 g
1 cup	OAT FLOUR	200 g
½ cup	WHOLEMEAL FLOUR, for batter	100 g
1 tsp	BAKING SODA	5 g
1 tbsp	FLAXSEED MEAL	15 g
2 tbsp	HOT WATER	30 ml
1 cup	SOY MILK	250 ml
Dash of	SALT	
2 tbsp	MAPLE SYRUP	30 ml
3 tbsp	SESAME SEEDS, toasted	45 g
½ cup	WHOLEMEAL FLOUR, to coat	100 g
1 tsp	CINNAMON POWDER, to coat	5 g
8 pc	PLANTAIN BANANAS or *sabá* bananas, halved sideways	160 g
	OLIVE OIL SPRAY	

(Serves 6)

Procedures:

1. Mix the flaxseed meal with the hot water and set aside to cool.
2. Cut the bananas in half, sideways, and set aside.
3. Mix the whole-meal flour with cinnamon powder and coat the plantain bananas with the mixture.

RECIPES AND COOKING NOTES

4. Put a cup of rolled oats in a blender and pulse until it turns into powder.
5. Mix the oats flour with the whole-meal flour and baking soda in a mixing bowl.
6. Add the smoothly mashed cavendish bananas together with the maple syrup and salt into the bowl with the flour mixture.
7. Add the soy milk and the flaxseed mixture with the above ingredients and mix until smooth.
8. Rest for five minutes to let the flours absorb the liquid and for it to form a steady consistency.
9. Heat a lightly sprayed non-stick frying pan to low heat.
10. In a small plate, separate some batter that is enough to cover a piece of plantain banana with it.
11. Using a large rubber scraper, drop on the prepared frying pan. Top with toasted sesame seeds.
12. Wait until the frying side of the battered banana is cooked well before turning to cook the other side with the sesame seeds.
13. Repeat until all bananas have been cooked.
14. Cool slightly before serving.

MEATLESS LÓNGGANÍSA PINÁIS

Ingredients:

1 recipe	MEATLESS LÓNGGANÍSA, recipe on p. 52	
3 cups	TURMERIC RICE, cooked	480 g
3 pc	TOMATOES, cut into wedges	270 g
Dash of	SALT	
	BANANA LEAVES, to wrap	
	TIE STRINGS	

(Serves 3)

SUSTAINING A PLANT-BASED DIET WITH FILIPINO FOOD

Procedures:

1. Divide the cooked lóngganísa from the referred recipe into three parts and set aside.
2. Wipe the banana leaves with a clean cloth and pass through an open fire to wilt and make the leaves pliant and soft prior to wrapping.
3. Lay a prepared banana leaf on a large plate and arrange a cup of rice, the lóngganísa and the lightly salted tomato wedges. The turmeric rice may be shaped manually to better manage the sealing of the parcel.
4. Repeat with another layer of banana leaf cover to secure the parcel prior to steaming. Tie up with a food-grade string. Do not use plastic or synthetic strings.
5. Preheat oven to 180°C or 360°F and arrange the banana parcels on a baking tray.
6. Bake for 15 minutes and turn off the heat but leave the parcels in the oven for another five minutes.
7. Take out of the oven and serve hot.

OVEN-ROASTED VEGETABLES WITH BEANS

Ingredients:

1 cup	SWEET POTATOES, diced into ¾-inch cubes	150 g
1 cup	BUTTERNUT PUMPKIN, diced into ¾-inch cubes	140 g
1 cup	CARROTS, diced into ¾-inch cubes	90 g
1 pack	SPICE MIX (Mexican Chipotle, Caldereta or Moroccan Seasoning)	57 g
1 cup	SNACK BEANS, recipe on p. 114	150 g

RECIPES AND COOKING NOTES

(Serves 3)

Procedures:

1. Preheat oven to 180°C, or 356°F.
2. In a mixing bowl, spread the seasonings evenly among mixed vegetables.
3. Line a baking tray with baking paper and arrange the diced vegetables.
4. Set the timer to thirty minutes but start watching out from twenty minutes of baking as cooking times vary for different ovens.
5. When done, take out of the oven and cool for five minutes in the baking tray before transferring to a serving plate.
6. Add the snack beans of choice, mix well and serve.

MIXED BEANS WITH BELL PEPPER GISÁDO

Ingredients:

1 cup	CANNED RED KIDNEY BEANS, rinsed and drained	170 g
1 cup	CANNED BLACK BEANS, rinsed and drained	170 g
1 cup	CANNED CANNELLINI BEANS, rinsed and drained	170 g
1 cup	CANNED CHICKPEAS, rinsed and drained	186 g
1 small pc	RED BELL PEPPER, diced	120 g
1 small pc	GREEN BELL PEPPER, diced	120 g
1 pc	ZUCCHINI, diced	170 g
1 pc	RED ONION, chopped	140 g
4 cloves	GARLIC, minced	16 g

SUSTAINING A PLANT-BASED DIET WITH FILIPINO FOOD

2 tbsp	SUNFLOWER OIL	30 g
¾ cup	HOT WATER	180 ml
½ pc	VEGETABLE STOCK CUBE	5 g
To taste,	SALT and PEPPER	

(Serves 4)

Procedures:

1. Dissolve the vegetable broth cube in hot water and set aside.
2. In a non-stick wok, heat the oil to medium heat.
3. Sauté the garlic until golden brown in color.
4. Add the onions just until they change colors.
5. Add the bell peppers and zucchini and continue mixing for two minutes.
6. Pour in the vegetable stock and wait until it boils.
7. Add the mixed beans and continue stirring in with the stock for five minutes.
8. Season with salt and pepper and cook for two more minutes before turning off the heat.

SQUASH SOUP WITH MORINGA LEAVES

Ingredients:

½ pc	SQUASH, steamed and pureed	500 g
½ cup, dry	YELLOW SPLIT PEAS, partially cooked for forty-five minutes	125 g
2 tbsp	SUNFLOWER OIL	30 ml
4 cloves	GARLIC, minced	16 g
1½ tsp	SEA SALT	8 g
Dash of	BLACK PEPPER	
1 pc	VEGETABLE STOCK CUBE	10 g
2 cups	WATER	500 g

RECIPES AND COOKING NOTES

1 cup	MORINGA or *malúnggay* leaves	45 g
½ cup	PEPPER LEAVES	10 g
½ cup	FRIED GARLIC, to serve	48 g
1 pc	RED ONION, chopped	120 g

(Serves 5)

Procedures:

1. Peel the squash and cut into small pieces.
2. Put enough water in a steamer boiler and boil to high heat.
3. Put in the squash pieces and boil for thirty minutes or until soft.
4. With a large blender puree the squash until smooth and set aside.
5. Clean and rinse the split peas in running water.
6. Transfer to a small cooking pot and add enough water to cover with an extra two inches above the peas.
7. Bring the pot to boil to medium heat.
8. When the water reaches a rolling boil, reduce heat to simmer for 45-50 minutes, adding water as necessary.
9. When cooked, set the peas aside and prepare to cook the soup.
10. Heat the oil in a cooking pot to medium heat.
11. Add the garlic and sauté until they turn golden brown in color.
12. Stir in the onions and continue cooking just until they change colors.
13. Pour in the water with the vegetable stock cube, add the sea salt and black pepper and bring to a boil.
14. Continue cooking until the cube is dissolved and has combined with the flavorings.
15. Add the squash puree, bring to a boil and add the cooked split peas.
16. Continue cooking for seven to ten more minutes or until the soup has reduced sufficiently and thickened.
17. Add the moringa and pepper leaves and turn off the heat.

SUSTAINING A PLANT-BASED DIET WITH FILIPINO FOOD

18. Serve with the fried garlic.

QUICK BANANA BLOSSOM SÍSIG

Ingredients:

1 can	BANANA BLOSSOM IN BRINE, drained	565 g
3 cloves	GARLIC, minced	12 g
1 pc	RED ONION, chopped	180 g
¼ cup	WHITE VINEGAR	60 ml
1 tbsp	VEGAN SHRIMP PASTE or VEGETARIAN MUSHROOM OYSTER SAUCE	15 ml
1 tbsp	SUNFLOWER OIL	15 ml
To taste,	SALT and PEPPER	

(Serves 2)

Procedures:

1. In a wire sieve, drain the canned banana blossoms and rinse in running water.
2. Press to expel any collected water and finely chop.
3. Heat the oil in a non-stick wok to medium heat and sauté the garlic until golden brown in color.
4. Add the onions and vegan shrimp paste just until the onions changed colors.
5. Stir in the vinegar and the chopped banana blossoms and continue stirring until everything is well absorbed by the vegetable.
6. Serve with raw onions.

RECIPES AND COOKING NOTES

RED CABBAGE COLESLAW WITH ATSÁRA PICKLING SOLUTION

Ingredients:

1 small pc	RED CABBAGE, chopped in small pieces	700 g
2 pc	RED ONIONS, chopped	300 g
10 cloves	GARLIC, whole	40 g
½ tbsp	COARSELY GROUND BLACK PEPPER	5 g
1 pc	CARROT, chopped	140 g
1 pc	RED BELL PEPPER, chopped	160 g
2 tbsp	GINGER, sliced thinly	70 g
1½ cup	COCONUT VINEGAR	375 ml
¾ cup	COCONUT SUGAR	180 g
2 tsp	SALT	10 g

Procedures:

1. In a small cooking pot, bring the coconut vinegar to a boil to low-medium heat.
2. Add the coconut sugar and stir just until it is completely melted.
3. Add the salt and mix before turning off the heat. Cool.
4. Chop all the coleslaw ingredients finely, except for the garlic and ginger.
5. In a large ceramic bowl, mix in all the vegetables and arrange well so that the garlic and ginger are positioned at the bottom.
6. Pour in the pickling solution and toss, making sure all the vegetables are well coated with the vinegar mixture.
7. Cover and chill in the refrigerator, tossing every two hours.

SUSTAINING A PLANT-BASED DIET WITH FILIPINO FOOD

BREADFRUIT AND GREEN BEANS IN COCONUT CREAM

Ingredients:

1 pc	RED ONION, halved lengthways and sliced thinly across	180 g
4 cloves	GARLIC, minced	16 g
2 tbsp	GINGER, cut into sticks	35 g
3 pc	SERRANO PEPPERS, sliced finely	2 g
4 pc	GREEN CHILLI PEPPERS, cut into ½-inch pieces	6 g
1 cup	CANNED COCONUT CREAM	250 ml
3 cups	GREEN BEANS, cut into one-inch pieces	300 g
1 can	BREADFRUIT IN BRINE	550 g
½ cup	WATER	125 ml
1 tbsp	VEGAN SHRIMP PASTE or VEGETARIAN MUSHROOM OYSTER SAUCE	15 ml
1 tbsp	SUNFLOWER OIL	15 ml

(Serves 4)

Procedures:

1. In a wire sieve, drain the canned breadfruit and rinse in running water.
2. Press to expel any collected liquid and finely chop the vegetable.
3. Heat the oil in a non-stick wok and sauté the garlic until golden brown in color.
4. Add the onions and ginger and cook until they change colors and release their aroma.
5. Add the coconut cream, water, peppers and vegan shrimp paste and bring to a boil.

RECIPES AND COOKING NOTES

6. Add in the green beans and breadfruit continue cooking for seven to ten minutes.
7. Taste and add seasonings as necessary.
8. Continue cooking until the coconut cream sauce is well reduced.
9. Turn off heat and rest for five minutes before serving.

VEGETABLE TINOLA

Ingredients:

2 tbsp	GINGER, crushed	30 g
1 pc	RED ONION, halved lengthways and sliced thinly across	160 g
4 cloves	GARLIC, minced	16 g
3 cups	WATER	750 ml
1½ pc	VEGETABLE STOCK CUBE, chicken-style	15 g
1 tbsp	VEGAN FISH SAUCE	15 g
½ pc	UNRIPE PAPAYA, peeled, pared and cut into 3-inch × ½-inch pieces	400 g
½ can	BAMBOO SHOOT HALVES, rinsed, drained and cut into 3-inch × ½-inch pieces	290 g
1 bundle	KANGKÓNG LEAVES, hard stems removed	300 g
1 cup	MORINGA LEAVES	45 g
1 block	FIRM TOFU, cut into 1½-inch cubes	250 g
Dash of	COARSELY GROUND BLACK PEPPER	
1 tbsp	SUNFLOWER OIL, to sauté	15 ml
¼ cup	SUNFLOWER OIL, to fry	60 ml

(Serves 4)

Procedures:

SUSTAINING A PLANT-BASED DIET WITH FILIPINO FOOD

1. Heat the oil in a frying pan to medium heat and fry the tofu pieces until they are golden brown in color. Drain of oil and pat dry with kitchen towels. Set aside.
2. In a large cooking pot, heat the oil to medium heat and sauté the garlic until golden brown in color.
3. Add the onions and ginger until they change colors and fragrant.
4. Increase heat and add the water, vegetable stock cubes, and seasonings and bring to a boil.
5. When the liquid reaches a rolling boil, reduce to simmer and leave to cook and let the flavors mix for ten to fifteen minutes.
6. Add the bamboo shoots and cook for another ten minutes.
7. Add the fried tofu and cook for another five minutes before adding the kangkóng leaves and moringa.
8. Turn off heat immediately after adding the green leaf vegetables.
9. Serve hot.

FREEZE-DRYING TOFU

Freeze the tofu, preferably overnight in the refrigerator. Thaw in advance when needed, until the tofu is as soft as it was before being frozen. Gently press on the tofu to expel as much water as possible and tap dry with kitchen towels. The result should be a tofu with firmer and meatier texture. It should be able to absorb at least twice as much liquid addition which makes it preferable for dishes that rely on sauces for taste.

RECIPES AND COOKING NOTES

TOFU KARÉ-KARÉ

Ingredients:

1 block	FIRM TOFU, freeze-dried, thawed and cut into 2-inch × 2-inch × 1-inch pieces	450 g
¼ cup	SUNFLOWER OIL, to fry	120 ml
1 tbsp	SUNFLOWER OIL, to sauté	15 ml
2 cups	STRING BEANS, cut into 2-inch long pieces	200 g
1 pc	BANANA BLOSSOM,	180 g
¼ cup	SALT, to prepare banana blossom	60 g
2 pc	EGGPLANT, cut diagonally into ½-inch thickness	170 g
3 pc	BOK CHOY, cleaned with leaves separated	100 g
3 cups	HOT WATER	375 ml
1½ pc	VEGETABLE STOCK CUBES, beef-style	15 g
¼ cup	RICE FLOUR, not the glutinous type	120 g
1 cup	PROTEIN PEANUT BUTTER	250 g
1 tsp	ANNATTO POWDER	5 g
4 cloves	GARLIC, minced	16 g
1 pc	RED ONION, halved lengthways and sliced thinly across	180 g
1 tbsp	VEGAN FISH SAUCE	15 ml
To taste,	SALT and PEPPER	

(Serves 5)

Procedures:

1. To prepare fresh banana blossom, please refer to Cooking Note on p. 81.

SUSTAINING A PLANT-BASED DIET WITH FILIPINO FOOD

2. Heat oil in a frying pan to medium heat and fry the tofu pieces until golden brown in color. Drain of oil and pat dry with kitchen towels. Set aside.
3. Dissolve the vegetable stock cubes in hot water and set aside.
4. Mix ½ cup of vegetable stock with the protein peanut butter and set aside.
5. In another bowl mix the annatto powder with ¼ cup of vegetable stock. Set aside.
6. Heat frying pan to medium heat and toast the rice flour until browned. Transfer to a bowl and add ½ cup of vegetable broth and mix well until it forms a paste. Set aside.
7. Put enough water in a steamer boiler and bring to a boil over high heat. When the water reaches a rolling boil, reduce heat to medium and fit in the steamer pan. Arrange the vegetables according to which could be taken out first.
8. When done, combine all the vegetables in a large mixing bowl and set aside.
9. in a large cooking pot, heat the oil to medium heat and sauté the garlic until golden brown in color.
10. Add the onions and cook just until they change colors.
11. Pour in the vegetable stock and bowl with the protein peanut butter mixture and cook for ten minutes.
12. Add the mixture with the annatto powder and cook for two more minutes.
13. Add the mixture with the rice flour paste, wait until it resumes to boil and reduce heat until slightly thick.
14. Pour in all of the vegetables all at once and wait until it boils again.
15. Season with vegan fish sauce and pepper. Add salt as necessary.
16. Add the fried tofu and reduce the sauce with more boiling until the sauce is sufficiently thick.
17. Rest in the heat source until ready to serve.

RECIPES AND COOKING NOTES

TOFU APRITÁDA

Ingredients:

1 block	FIRM TOFU, freeze-dried, thawed and cut into 2-inch × 2-inch × 1-inch pieces	300 g
4 cloves	GARLIC, minced	16 g
1 pc	RED ONION, halved lengthways and sliced thinly across	180 g
1 cup	TOMATO SAUCE	250 ml
1 cup	HOT WATER	250 g
½ pc	VEGETABLE STOCK CUBE, chicken-style	10 g
¼ cup	SUNFLOWER OIL, to fry	120 g
1 tbsp	SUNFLOWER OIL, to sauté	15 ml
1 cup	FROZEN GREEN PEAS, thawed and parboiled	110 g
2 cups	GREEN BEANS, cut into 2-inch pieces	200 g
1 pc	CARROT, sliced into 1-inch lengths	160 g
2 cups	SWEET POTATOES, cut into 1½-inch cubes	320 g
To taste,	SALT and PEPPER	
1 tbsp	COCONUT SUGAR	15 g

(Serves 3)

Procedures:

1. Heat the oil in a frying pan to medium heat and fry the freeze-dried tofu pieces until golden brown in color. Drain of oil and pat dry with kitchen towels.
2. Heat enough water with some salt in a small cooking pot to medium heat.

SUSTAINING A PLANT-BASED DIET WITH FILIPINO FOOD

3. When the water reaches a rolling boil, reduce heat to simmer and add the frozen peas.
4. Boil for five minutes and drain in a wire sieve when done.
5. Heat the oil in a cooking pot to medium heat and sauté the garlic until golden brown in color.
6. Add the onions and cook just until they change colors.
7. Add the water, vegetable stock cube and tomato sauce and wait until it begins to boil.
8. Add the carrot pieces and the cubed sweet potato and cook for fifteen minutes.
9. Add the green beans and cook for another seven minutes.
10. Add the fried tofu pieces and the green peas and cook for another three minutes before turning off the heat.
11. Rest for five minutes before serving.

TOFU SKEWERS

Ingredients:

Marinade:

3 pc	LEMON, juiced	300 g
7 cloves	GARLIC, minced	28 g
½ cup	TAMARI	120 ml
1 tbsp	GINGER, crushed	15 g
8 tbsp	COCONUT SUGAR	120 g
1 tbsp	SUNFLOWER OIL	15 ml
4 pc	SERRANO PEPPERS, sliced thinly	2 g
Dash of	COARSELY GROUND BLACK PEPPER	

Barbecue:

2 blocks	FIRM TOFU, freeze-dried, thawed and cut into 1-inch cubed pieces	900 g

RECIPES AND COOKING NOTES

10 pc   BAMBOO SKEWERS

(Serves 5)

Procedures:

1. Make sure the water content of the freeze-dried tofu has been sufficiently expelled.
2. Once cut into the suggested size, marinate the tofu pieces overnight.
3. When ready to cook, prepare the tofu pieces by sticking into the skewers and set aside.
4. Transfer the marinade into a small cooking pot.
5. Add ½ cup water and bring to a boil over medium heat.
6. When the marinade mix begins to boil, reduce heat to low and reduce the marinade until it is of spreading consistency, but taking care not to let it burn.
7. Prepare the hot coals, elevate the grill and start cooking the tofu skewers.
8. As soon as they start heating up, baste the tofu skewers with the reduced marinade until cooked.

BANANA BLOSSOM LITSÓN PAKSÍW

Ingredients:

1 block	FIRM TOFU, freeze-dried, thawed and cut into 2-inch × 2-inch × 1-inch pieces	300 g
1 can	BANANA BLOSSOM IN BRINE, drained	565 g
½ tbsp	SUNFLOWER OIL, to sauté	8 ml
¼ cup	SUNFLOWER OIL, to fry	60 ml
1 pc	RED ONION, halved lengthways and cut thinly across	140 g

145

SUSTAINING A PLANT-BASED DIET WITH FILIPINO FOOD

6 cloves	GARLIC, crushed	24 g
½ cup	COCONUT VINEGAR	125 ml
¾ cup	WATER	180 ml
1 bottle	LITSÓN SAUCE	375 g
6 tbsp	COCONUT SUGAR	90 g
2 tsp	CINNAMON POWDER	10 g
2 pc	BAY LEAVES	
¼ cup	BREAD CRUMBS	60 g
½ pc	VEGETABLE STOCK CUBE, chicken-style	5 g
To taste,	SALT AND PEPPER	

(Serves 4)

Procedures:

1. Make sure the water content of the freeze-dried tofu has been sufficiently expelled.
2. Heat oil in a frying pan to medium heat and fry the tofu pieces until lightly brown in color. Set aside.
3. In a wire sieve, drain the canned banana blossoms and rinse in running water.
4. Press to expel any collected water and finely chop. Set aside.
5. Heat the oil in a cooking pot to medium heat and sauté the garlic until golden brown in color.
6. Add the sliced onion and cook just until they change colors.
7. Add the vinegar, water and the vegetable stock cube, litsón sauce and bring to a boil, uncovered, and continue boiling for five minutes. Thicken with the bread crumbs.
8. Add the bay leaves, ground cinnamon, sugar and banana blossoms and leave to cook for ten minutes.
9. Add the fried tofu pieces and continue to cook for two minutes before turning off the heat.

RECIPES AND COOKING NOTES

FREEZE-DRIED TOFU ESKABÉTSE

Ingredients:

1 block	FIRM TOFU, freeze-dried, thawed and cut into 2-inch × 2-inch × 1-inch cubes	300 g
1 pc	RED ONION, halved lengthways and sliced thinly across	180 g
1 pc	GREEN BELL PEPPER, julienned	200 g
1 pc	RED BELL PEPPER, julienned	200 g
1 tbsp	GINGER, cut into matchstick pieces	15 g
4 cloves	GARLIC, minced	16 g
Pinch of	COARSELY GROUND BLACK PEPPER	
¼ cup	SUNFLOWER OIL, to fry	60 ml
2 tbsp	SUNFLOWER OIL, to sauté	30 g
5 tbsp	DARK SOY SAUCE	75 ml
5 tbsp	COCONUT VINEGAR	75 ml
4 tbsp	COCONUT SUGAR	60 g
2 tbsp	CORNSTARCH	30 g
2 tbsp	WATER, for cornstarch	30 ml
¾ cup	WATER	180 ml

(Serves 3)

Procedures:

1. Make sure the water content of the freeze-dried tofu has been sufficiently expelled.
2. Heat oil in a frying pan to medium heat and fry the tofu pieces until lightly brown in color. Set Aside.
3. In a small mixing bowl mix water, vinegar, sugar and cornstarch.
4. In a non-stick wok, heat oil to medium heat and sauté the garlic until golden brown in color.
5. Add the sliced onions and the ginger and cook until soft and fragrant.

147

SUSTAINING A PLANT-BASED DIET WITH FILIPINO FOOD

6. Add the bell peppers and cook until soft.
7. Pour in the liquid mixture and cook while constantly stirring until it forms a slightly thick sauce. Turn off heat.
8. Arrange the tofu pieces in a platter and pour in the sauce.

TOFU SÍSIG

Ingredients:

2 block	FIRM TOFU, freeze-dried, thawed and cut into ½-inch cubes	600 g
1 pc	RED ONION, chopped	180 g
4 cloves	GARLIC, minced	16 g
¼ cup	SUNFLOWER OIL, to fry	60 ml
1 tbsp	SUNFLOWER OIL, to sauté	15 ml
2 pc	SERRANO PEPPERS	2 g
2 pc	GREEN CHILLI PEPPERS	4 g
1 tbsp	VEGETARIAN MUSHROOM OYSTER SAUCE	15 ml
½ tbsp	LIGHT SOY SAUCE	8 ml
¼ cup	VEGAN MAYONNAISE	60 g
1 pc	LEMON, juiced	120 g

(Serves 4)

Procedures:

1. Make sure the water content of the freeze-dried tofu has been sufficiently expelled and cut the tofu into required size.
2. In a non-stick wok, heat oil to medium heat and fry the tofu pieces by constantly stirring until they form a light golden crust. Drain and set aside.

RECIPES AND COOKING NOTES

3. In a separate wok, heat oil to medium heat and sauté the garlic until golden brown in color.
4. Add the onion pieces and cook just until they change colors.
5. Add the tofu pieces and chillies, toss and mix well.
6. Season with vegetarian mushroom oyster sauce and light soy sauce and continue cooking for two more minutes.
7. Turn off heat and add the vegan mayonnaise and mix thoroughly.
8. Add in the lemon juice just before serving.

ACKNOWLEDGEMENT

Our heartfelt gratitude to **Sarah Alberto** of You Tube's *Doodles by Sarah* for unselfishly helping us out with the artwork during the conceptual phase of this book up until its first versions.

We also acknowledge with our sincere thanks artist splinex from VectorStock® for the rice field image on the current front cover of this book.

DEDICATION

This book is dedicated to the memory of my mother, **INANG PURING**, and to my mother-in-law, **NANAY CONSOLING,** who is recovering from the amputation of a second limb in eleven months.

These two most important and irreplaceable people in our life had to be among thousands of unnecessary victims of the completely expendable condition called adult-onset diabetes.

It is our prayer that tragedies such as these could be lessened with our better sharing of meaningful information, knowing as we do that we are all in this together.

BIBLIOGRAPHY

Scott, William Henry. *Barangay: Sixteenth Century Philippine Culture and Society.* Ateneo de Manila University Press, Quezon City, Philippines. 1994.

Agoncillo, Teodoro A. *History Of The Filipino People, Eighth Edition.* Quezon City, Philippines. 1990.

Almario, Virgilio S., Chief Editor. *UP Diksiyonaryong Filipino.* Pasig City, Philippines. 2001.

Alvina, Corazon S. "Regional Dishes". *The Food of the Philippines: Authentic Recipes From the Pearl of the Orient.* Reynaldo G. Alejandro, et al. Hongkong. 1999.

Blair, Emma Helen and Robertson, James Alexander. *The Philippine Islands 1493-1898, Volume XXXIII—1519-1522.* Cleveland, Ohio. 1916.

Nolledo, Wilfrido D. *But For The Lovers.* Normal, Illinois. 1970.

McGee, Harold. *On Food & Cooking: An Encyclopedia Of Kitchen Science, History And Culture.* London, Great Britain. 2004.

Shurtleff, William & Aoyagi Akiko. *The Book Of Tofu: Protein Source of the Future—Now!* New York, United States of America. 1979.

Fenix, Michaela., Editor. *Kulinarya: A Guidebook To Philippine Cuisine.* Mandaluyong City, Philippines. 2013.

Fernandez, Doreen G. "The Food World of Miguel Ruiz." *Reflections on Philippine Culture and Society: Festschrift in Honor of William Henry Scott.* Jesus T. Peralta, Editor. Ateneo de Manila University Press. Quezon City, Philippines. 2001.

Fernandez, Doreen G. "What is Filipino Food?" *The Food of the Philippines: Authentic Recipes From The Pearl of the Orient.* Reynaldo G. Alejandro, et al. Hongkong. 1999.

Fernandez, Doreen G. "The Filipino Fiesta". *The Food of the Philippines: Authentic Recipes From The Pearl of the Orient.* Reynaldo G. Alejandro, et al. Hongkong. 1999.

Mindell, Earl with Hester Mundis, *Earl Mindell's New Vitamin Bible, Revised and Updated.* New York. 2011.

Greger, Michael with Gene Stone. *How Not To Die.* London, U.K. 2018.

Barnard, Neal D. *Power Foods For The Brain.* New York. 2013.

Fuhrman, Joel, M.D. *The End Of Diabetes.* New York. 2013.

RECIPE INDEX

Ampalayá Smoothie, 120
Bamboo Shoot Adóbo, 89
Bamboo Shoot Gisádo, 92
Banana Blossom Litsón Paksíw, 145
Banana Blossom with Sótanghón, 84
Banana Oats Maruyà, 130
Barbecue Broad Beans and Chickpeas, 108
Bitter Gourd Tomato Ensaladá, 104
Bitter Gourd with Black Beans Gisádo, 53
Braised Carrots and Chayote, 123
Breadfruit and Green Beans in Coconut Cream, 138
Bok Choy and Tofu Gisádo, 50
Boiled Brown Rice, 32
Boiled Brown Rice, 35
Brown Rice Arroz Caldo, 40
Brown Rice Brínghe, 38
Brown Rice with Quinoa, 37
Cabbage and Carrots Gisádo, 93
Canned Beans Snacks, 113
Carrots and Green Beans Ensaladá, 102
Cauliflower Ensaladá, 103
Cheesy Oats Púto, 126
Cheesy Pimiento Spread, 87
Creamed Corn-Split Pea Suwám, 121
Crispy-Fried Tofu with Vinegar Dip, 47
Eggplant Bisték, 95
Eggplant Iníhaw with Coconut Milk, 86
Ensaladáng Pilipino, 99
Freeze-dried Tofu Eskabétse, 147
Green Beans with Tofu Gisádo, 48
Kale and White Bean Dip, 57
Kale Chips, 54
Kale Quinoa Ensaladá, 69

155

Kangkóng Adóbo, 88
Laíng, 97
Laksá-Laksá, 78
Leafy greens with Stir-fry Sauce, 96
Lentil and Sweet Potato Bóla-Bóla, 122
Lima Beans Sinigáng, 109
Lima beans with Sweet Potato Gisádo, 111
Lumpiyâ Plate, 65
Lumpiyâng Prito, 67
Mango Cucumber Ensaladá, 68
Meatless Longganísa, 61
Meatless Longganísa Pináis, 131
Mixed Beans with Bell Pepper Gisádo, 133
Mung Bean Sprouts Ensaladá, 101
Mung Beans with Bitter Gourd Leaves Gisádo, 90
Mung Beans with Maple Soy Milk, 129
Mushroom and Bok Choy Gisádo, 94
Ókoy, 70
Oven-Roasted Vegetables with Beans, 132
Oven-Roasted Vegetables with Garden Ensaladá, 106
Oyster Mushroom Gisádo 85
Pasta with Tomato Pesto, 116
Pesto Pizza, 116
Picadillo with Sweet Potatoes and Sabá, 62
Pico de Gallo, 100
Pinakbét, 72
Red Cabbage Coleslaw with Atsára Pickling Solution, 137
Roasted Lima Beans Snack, 119
Salabát, 127
Snake Beans Adóbo, 87
Sótanghón Asado Noodles, 82
Sótanghón Gisádo, 76
Sótanghón Hot Pot, 80
Sótanghón with Bottle Gourd, 77
Sótanghón with Sponge Gourd, 81
Spaghetti with Sweet Tomato Sauce, 124
Spicy Tofu Pináis, 52
Squash Soup with Moringa Leaves, 134

Staple Bowl, 44
Stir-fried Mixed Vegetables, 63
Stir-fried Pinakbét Vegetables, 74
Tahô with Tapioca Pearls, 95
Tápa Bits Pináis with Turmeric Rice, 128
Tápa Bits Toppings, 59
Toasted Brown Rice, 42
Tofu Apritáda, 143
Tofu Bisték, 46
Tofu Karékaré, 141
Tofu Paksíw with lily Blossoms, 49
Tofu Sísig, 148
Tofu Skewers, 144
Tofu with Garlic Leaves Gisádo, 51
Tofu-Taro Siomai, 57
Tomato Basil Pesto, 114
Turmeric Brown Rice, 36
Quick Banana Blossom Sísig, 136
Vegetable Tinóla, 139
White Beans with Tomato Pesto, 115

ABOUT THE AUTHOR

The author turned to purely plant-based eating more than three years ago and averted what would certainly have been a downhill slide towards a diabetic condition.

Aside from being a meticulous home cook, he took a course in commercial baking twenty-six years ago and has been baking since.

He was a community organizer, technical writer, project officer, university researcher, development worker for a non-government organization, project evaluator and middle manager in charge of policy of a nationwide business lending program of a government agency in the Philippines before coming to live permanently in Australia with his wife and two daughters.

He was born and raised in Pampanga and educated in Manila where he studied journalism and political science. His interests include history, literature, organic agriculture and container food crop gardening.

Made in the USA
Monee, IL
26 October 2023